MY

A TO Z

OF LIVING WITH

ASPERGER'S SYNDROME

AND

AUTISM

BY LYNNE WATKINS

Copyright

©2013 Lynne Watkins

All rights reserved. No part of this publication may be reproduced, stored in a retrieval system, or transmitted, in any form or by any means without the prior written permission of the author, nor otherwise circulated in any form of binding or cover than that in which it is published and without a similar condition being imposed on the subsequent purchaser.

ISBN: 978-1-291-29411-8

This book is dedicated to my children, Brynmor and Rhodri, who are unable to understand the contents, but without them it could not have been written.

Also to all those adults and children who have been included in the narratives within. Having taken pains to preserve their anonymity, I am unable to mention them individually here.

Also grateful thanks to Dr Peter Carpenter, who diagnosed my Asperger's Syndrome in 2001, and who agreed to write the foreword to this book. This helped me realise that it will hopefully be useful to those struggling to understand people with an autistic spectrum condition.

Contents:

Foreword	1
Preface	3
What is Autism/Asperger's Syndrome	5
A is for Apology	15
B is for Being Different	21
C is for Conversation	25
D is for Daydreams	35
E is for Eye Contact	37
F is for Friends	41
G is for Growing Up	47
H is for Hell	49
I is for Imagination	53
J is for July	55
K is for Keep Hoping	57
L is for Letters	61

M is for Meltdowns	67
N is for Normal	73
O is for Organisation	75
P is for Prosopagnosia	79
Q is for Questions	81
R is for Routines & Rules	87
S is for Sensitivities	97
T is for Treating People like Parcels	103
U is for Understanding	107
V is for Vitamins and Diet	117
W is for Worrying	123
X is for Xmas	125
Y is for You	129
Z is for Zzzz	133
The End and The Future	137

FOREWORD

I first met Lynne, Bryn and Rhodri about 20 years ago. At the time I was surprised to find how Lynne was surviving and staying apparently sane with her house looking like a building site due to the activities of her sons and with her life so dominated by them. Two extremely different sons, both with autism but with very different personalities and individual needs.

Over the years Lynne has stayed sane, and pushed and pulled her two sons though childhood and adolescence to adulthood. Her sons have grown up and she has again developed a life for herself. It has not been easy, sometimes due to the reactions of others around her. It has however had its rewards and delights for all of them.

In this book Lynne has not written her life story. She has illustrated her experiences. It is full of anecdotes and pragmatic solutions, written with the insight of someone with autism observing and managing her children with autism. It is written with humour and with a painful honesty.

I enjoyed reading this book and have dipped back into it several times. I have found myself drawn back to it. I learnt more about the experience of autism and more ideas on how to solve problems. I also learnt that whilst life has its frightening times, one can succeed.

Dr Peter Carpenter   F.R.C.Psych.
Consultant Psychiatrist Intellectual Disabilities.
July 2012

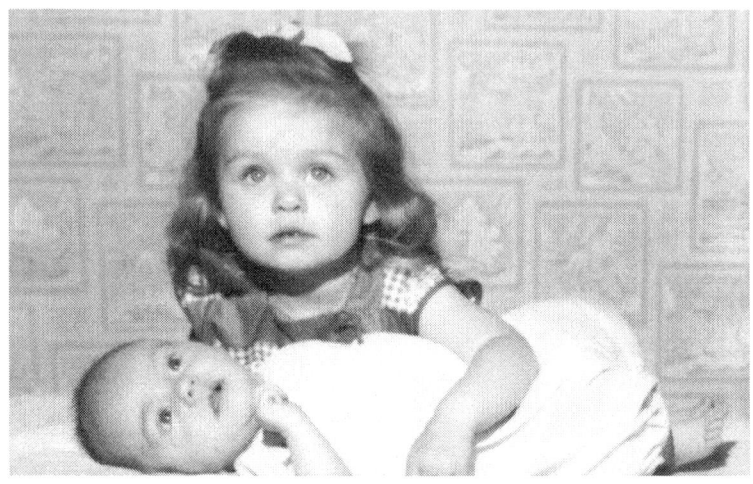

This is a photograph of me in 1962, aged 2 years old. My Mum tells me that at that time I was very protective of my baby brother. I used to tell everyone who came to the house that they had to come to see him, and woke him up to see them! This didn't please him or my mum much! It seems I was a chatterbox at that time, I wonder when I started to lose the ability to talk to people.
(See C for Communication)

PREFACE

My family i.e. my children and I have all been diagnosed as having an autistic spectrum disorder. Brynmor (born 1989) was diagnosed with autism and learning difficulties aged 3½ years. Rhodri (born 1991) was diagnosed with learning difficulties aged 2½ years. Although generally referred to as being autistic from this time, he did not have an official autism diagnosis on his statement of special educational needs until he was about 6 years old. This is despite being in the autistic class at school, where he started a week before his third birthday. Professionals kept telling me that it was not possible to have two autistic children, as the condition was not genetic. I think this view may have changed in later years, as there are many families where more than one sibling has autism.

This book is a collection of my ideas on Autism and Asperger's Syndrome. I like routines and patterns. It has been written in the pattern of the alphabet. I seem to spend a lot of time telling people who I meet, about my children and myself, the things we find difficult and how we have found a way round our difficulties. Between the chapters, I have problem solving ideas, including information on websites where to buy the materials required.

I wanted to write this book, so others may learn about the problems and may find how to act around autistic people, and perhaps to consider their own thoughts about the condition. Of course, I don't know if all my problems are due to the autism, or are 'just me'. Other people may have different ideas about autism. However, in this book I wish to explain what it's like to be me.

All the suggestions in this book are my own ideas. I am not medically qualified, but have over 50 years experience of living with and supporting others who are on the autistic spectrum. Please speak to a medical professional before following any advice or suggestions from this book.

All people on the autistic spectrum are not the same, in the way that no two NT (Neuro-typical / non-autistic) people are the same. So the ideas in this book will not work for everyone, but may be worth a try.

In this book, I have only named my children, and people who agreed to have their real name included, or who have died. I hope that other individuals are described in a way that they are unable to be identified.

What is Autism / Asperger's Syndrome?

A Typical Dictionary definition:

Autism = a mental condition characterised by great difficulty in communicating with others and in using language and abstract concepts

Asperger's Syndrome = a mild autistic disorder characterized by awkwardness in social interaction, pedantry in speech, and preoccupation with very narrow interests.

For years, the dictionary definition used to describe Autism as a condition affecting children. I'm glad to see that it has been updated as I always wondered what happened to these children when they became adults!

Autism is a very large spectrum of disabilities. It includes Asperger's Syndrome, which is sometimes called "High Functioning Autism", although my letter of diagnosis mentions "A-typical Autism" and "Asperger's Syndrome". It is named after Hans Asperger, an Austrian psychiatrist and paediatrician, who first published work about the syndrome in 1944 and had many of the symptoms himself. However, it was not recognised as a diagnosis in the UK until the 1990's (when I was in my thirties!).

This has led to many adults not being diagnosed, and as people with Asperger's Syndrome are normally very intelligent, many people with the condition may be in very responsible jobs. Most people have met doctors, professors etc with no social skills but who are very skilled at their profession.

Some of the problems associated with the syndrome are:

Lack of empathy
Little ability to form friendships
One-sided conversations
Intense absorption in a special interest

Hans Asperger called children with the condition "little professors". I think I was lucky that Asperger's Syndrome was not recognised when I was young. I was intelligent and learned to cope with the problems, to hide them from the outside world, and just to get on with life as it was thrown at me. I'm concerned about children today that are informed from an early age that they have 'special needs' and given a variety of diagnoses. I remember when I worked at a youth club for young people with special needs. Several teenagers were sat round discussing their diagnoses e.g. Asperger's, ADHD (Attention Deficit Hyperactivity Disorder), NCD (Non Compliance Disorder) and several other initials, some of which were new to me. As I entered the room, one called to me "What have you got?" I replied I had Asperger's Syndrome and Triple-X Syndrome, and there was silence for a few seconds with surprise. Although they knew me well, the subject of my diagnosis hadn't been discussed before. I had to explain yes, I drive, I have a house, children, a job ... – having Asperger's Syndrome doesn't make me incapable of having a reasonably normal life.

In case you are wondering, at this point, Triple-X means having three X chromosomes, instead of the normal two. I was only informed I had this when I had a blood test to find out if I had a chromosome abnormality that could have been passed to my sons. This wasn't what they were testing for, but they said "by the way did you know you had Triple-X syndrome?". I didn't, but as the symptoms include a lack of social skills, I seem to have acquired this difficulty twice.

I have always been surprised at the large number of children and teenagers with Asperger's, ADHD etc who I have met in the course of my work, who inform me that they are 'special', that I can't 'tell them off' because they have special needs.

The following is a sample conversation, and one I particularly remember.

'Jeff' (12 yr old boy with Asperger's) is throwing balls at 'Sally' (similar aged girl with physical & learning difficulties) in a soft play area. The plastic balls hurt when thrown at someone with force, and the girl wasn't able to move quickly due to her disabilities.

I stood between them, to block balls being picked up and thrown again.

Me: "stop doing that, you are hurting Sally"

Jeff: "You can't stop me I can do what I like, I have special needs."

Me: "Well, I'm not going to let you continue hurting Sally, so please leave the soft play area and go and do something else."

Jeff: "You can't tell me off. My mum says I have to tell teachers that you can't tell me off. I have Asperger's Syndrome and I can do what I want."

Me: "I have Asperger's Syndrome too, so that must mean I can do what I want, and I want you to leave the soft play area NOW."

Jeff is flummoxed by the logic of this, as his mother hasn't primed him with an answer to this one. He leaves the area.

I was left wondering if Jeff's mother actually understands the effect of her words on her son. Does she really think he should be allowed to go around hurting other children at will?

What will come of these children when they become adults?

"I can drive through a red traffic light because I have Asperger's."?? "I can steal from you, because I can do what I want."?? No wonder they say the prisons are full of people with ADHD/Asperger's Syndrome!

I hope that it is only the minority of parents who teach this to their children. 'Jeff' came from an educated family, and had a high IQ.

I have read school reports of children with Asperger's Syndrome, in mainstream schools, who can 'choose' whether to do the work that the rest of the class have to do, who get rewards of fruit and computer time if they do the work done by everyone else, but the rest of the class don't get a reward, only them.

I don't see how this is integration, to put these children on a pedestal, to give them their own way all the time, to encourage them to be different and to therefore be a victim of bullying. I can quite see why other children in the class would resent a child who gets all these 'rewards' that they don't, who has a support assistant to do his writing for him (it's usually a 'him'), and who can choose whether he has to do as he is told. The result is a lot of spoilt, unruly children who are not encouraged to fit into the world.

Particularly worrying to me, is the young children who go to their own reviews. My children were unable to sit still more than three minutes, if that, and didn't attend. Those that do, hear parents, teachers and other professionals discussing how they are unable to socialise, unable to do this, that and the other …. I know, from experience, that I will always believe what I am told. If my mother says "you can't do that" then I will believe her and 'know' I am unable to do the task.

How much better it would be if children were encouraged to think positively and know they can socialise etc, then they would have the confidence to try. Hearing something like "he always hits other children when the bell sounds", will only ingrain the action into his brain and he will continue to hit in this situation. Of course these problems need to be discussed, as they have been for my sons, but surely not in the hearing of the children concerned.

The undiagnosed adults of today, like me, just got on with things and did the work, because we were punished if we didn't. Many now have good qualifications and jobs. These children of today will not have this, they will be having 'support' for most of their lives, due to not learning to cope with life at an early age.

This "I have special needs" syndrome, only affects children at mainstream schools. Those at special needs schools are not taught this 'syndrome', as all the children have special needs. The result is that these children are mainly polite, well behaved and a good deal easier to communicate with, as they haven't spent most of their lives being told they are 'special'.

Autism at the other end of the spectrum is associated with severe learning difficulties. Both my sons are at this end of the spectrum. These adults and children often have no, or very little, speech, very little understanding of the outside world, and a great deal of frustration at not being able to make themselves understood. They may have what is termed 'challenging behaviour'. What is actually understood by this term varies depending on to whom you speak.

I went to a talk about dealing with challenging behaviour some years ago. It was meant for teachers, but the local autistic society was given some tickets to give parents and I went along as I was having a lot of problems with Rhodri. At question time, one teacher got up and said there was a child with challenging behaviour in her class. When asked what form this behaviour took, she said he kept throwing his pencil on the floor and she didn't know what to do about it. There was silence round the room, as most of us wished this was all we had to cope with! Rhodri was having a very difficult period while he had a problem with gluten (see chapter V for Vitamins and Diet), and I was being attacked by him regularly.

Challenging behaviour, in whatever form it takes, is normally due to frustration. This is especially the case for children, and adults, who have no or limited communication. Although, even those who can talk, are often unable to express themselves in order to be understood. (See chapter 'C for communication).

I often tell people "imagine you are at the dentist, your mouth is propped open with that item that dentists use to stop you closing your mouth. The dentist and his assistant are having a conversation over your head, talking about you, and saying something wrong. You are desperate to tell them, but unable to speak. Now, in this situation you wait until the end and say "By the way, about what you were saying ....", but just imagine never being able to give your view, to correct what people saying, to say what you want or need. Never being able to say you have a headache, you are hot/cold, you don't like certain foods you keep being given. This is what it is like for these autistic people like my sons."

I was astounded when I read recently that "challenging behaviour in people with learning difficulties is the result of abuse or bad parenting". Let me assure you that is not the case, it is caused by frustration and lack of understanding.

Someone once said to me "When you see an autistic child, look at the father". This is because autism, like many learning difficulties, is usually recognised in more boys than girls, and is passed down in families. Any special needs school, residential home etc, will have more boys than girls. In my case, of course, it's look at the mother! I have two autistic sons, now aged 21 and 23. Autism seems to get 'worse' as it is passed down the generations. I believe that the world we now live in has accentuated the problems.

I personally believe that although autism is passed down through families, something happens to trigger it to a level where it may cause problems. Every time I try to describe the problems I (or my children) have because we are autistic, I get the reaction "but I do that too, so that can't be autism" to at least one of the problems. Other people's "I do that" generally relate to different things I am saying. But I do all the problems and others may only do one or two. So, everyone has a 'bit' of autism in them, but those diagnosed have all the 'bits'. I think my triple-X may have been my 'trigger'. I believe the MMR vaccine caused my children's learning difficulties and digestive problems, although I know that their autism was passed down to them from me. I believe that Bryn was fortunate that he kept being ill and didn't have his MMR until he was over 2 years old, so he was talking before he had it. He lost his speech after the vaccination, but later learned to vocalise after Auditory Integration Therapy.

Rhodri was given his MMR at 12 months before he was talking, and he has never spoken. Rhodri also had the booster at 3, even though I had signed the form to say that I refused permission. I didn't find this out until he was 12, as the school didn't tell me at the time and it was too late to put in a complaint to the health authority which has to be done within 8 years from the incident. I was told that he was given it as I had agreed with a health visitor that he could have it.

A health visitor <u>had</u> visited me at home, and I finally agreed verbally to him having the vaccination, as she refused to leave my house until I did, but I believed that what I later wrote on the form and signed would take precedence, but apparently not. So Rhodri ended up with a double dose, and will cost the country many thousands of pounds in support fees for the rest of his life.

On the positive side, people with Asperger's Syndrome and Autism are normally:
>
> Truthful
> Punctual
> Intelligent
> Dedicated
> Logical Thinking
> Have A Good Memory.

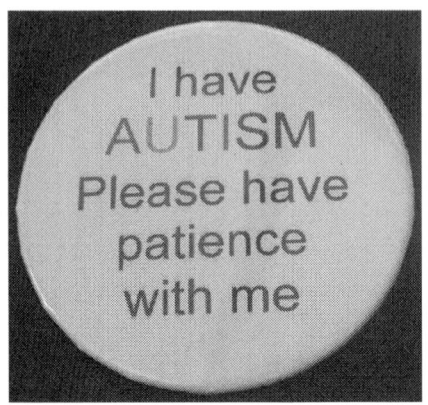

One of the badges I made for Bryn to wear when he was younger, so that people would understand that he was autistic. The AUTISM was printed in rainbow colours. See page 17

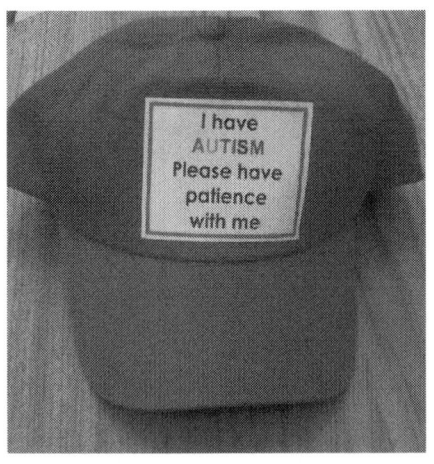

Rhodri preferred to wear a cap. He always refused to wear badges.

A IS FOR APOLOGY

It's often said that people with Asperger's Syndrome don't do 'grey', it's either black or white. I seem to spend a lot of time apologising, as unintentionally I have upset someone. I often say what I think, which can get me into trouble. Having said that, I learnt as a small child that if someone asks, "does this look nice?" I was to say "yes", whether it did or not.

Other rules were:

Always say "thank you, that's nice", for gifts, even if you didn't like them.
Always say "no, thank you" if offered food, in case you looked greedy.
Never ask, wait to be asked. (when due to the rule above I usually had to say no).
Do as you are told
Always agree, it keeps people happy.
Leave things as you find them.
Mind your own business – don't tell other people when they do things wrong.
Don't interrupt when someone is talking.

Doing as you are told, often also causes problems, because most autistic people take things literally. The old example is of the doctors' receptionist who says "take a seat" and the patient, who picks up the chair, and says "take it where?"

I'm also always apologising on my sons' behalf, and having to explain that they are autistic, when they have done something wrong. This includes putting out a hand as they walk along, which often touches people as they pass. Which almost led to Bryn (aged about 5) being hit by a man with a walking stick – his hand touched the man as we walked past, and thinking he was being assaulted, he lashed out – I moved Bryn just in time! Now, some people get worried when faced by a six foot 23 year old, leaping up & down and hand flapping, because he is excited.

I'm reminded of my son in a local shop, he was wandering round while I was looking at something. There was a noise to my right, and I looked round calling "Bryn", and the goods lift opened. A woman came out, and asked Bryn, "Did you press the button", Bryn said "yes", she was obviously nonplussed, having expected him to deny it, and just said, "Well don't do it again!".

Having Asperger's Syndrome, and needing to keep to rules myself, I get worried when things are 'wrong'. I have naturally got used to being with two children with severe learning difficulties and autism, however, sometimes get annoyed by other people's reactions to them.

One elderly woman complained about the noise Rhodri (aged 10) was making in the supermarket queue – he was actually standing still, and making his 'happy' noise, waiting unusually patiently for his turn – I told her, that he was autistic, that I would love him to talk, but he couldn't, that this was his happy noise, and if she didn't like that, it was lucky he wasn't making his unhappy one!! She said she hadn't known anything was wrong with him – a poor excuse due to his size and he was wearing a harness, with dog lead attached! I found that harnesses & reins, like those intended for toddlers, didn't have a long enough rein. I preferred to be able to be further away from him, if he was in a biting mood, and a dog lead was just right to attach to the harness. I couldn't let him walk on his own as he would run away, and had no idea of stopping at roads, and if I held his hand it was easier for him to bite me.

"I'm sorry, he's autistic" was getting to be a continual saying for me, so I made some badges that said "I have AUTISM, please have patience with me". This seemed to solve some problems and many people noticed the badge and were helpful. I'm often told by other parents that they keep meeting people who have never heard of, or know anyone with, autism. I'm not sure where they go to see these people. These days, I find most people know someone. I'm always being told "my neighbour's son has..", "my friend's brother's son has ...." etc.

When Bryn was first diagnosed it was a different story. This was in 1993, when he was three and a half. At that time our GP said he had "never seen an autistic child before", although what he meant was he had never seen one who was diagnosed – due to the number of undiagnosed autistics that must have been around at the time.

The same went for social workers and health visitors. I had a collection of information leaflets from the National Autistic Society and some computer printouts. I was contacted several times by local health or social workers, who had heard that I had autistic children and were told that I would provide them with an 'information pack' they could give to parents. This continued until I moved to another area. Later, the health authority handed out 'information packs' to parents of newly diagnosed autistics, and seemed to think that it was their own idea!

After Rhodri was diagnosed autistic, I was pointed out at the local National Autistic Society group as "the one who has two". This is not uncommon these days, but at that time we only knew of one other person (in another county) who "had two" (autistic children).

What always irritates me is the T-shirt produced by an Autism society which has "I'm not naughty, I'm Autistic" printed on the front. This seems to be saying that autistic children are never naughty. I assure you that, like all children, they can be naughty. That is, they know they are doing wrong, as opposed to not knowing.

As an example, Rhodri would wait until someone turned their back for an instant before making his move to escape, climbing a six foot fence with ease. He knew exactly what he was doing was wrong or he would not have waited for his carer to turn away. What he did not understand was the reason that he shouldn't go out, was that he had no sense of road danger and would be in collision with a car in a very short time.

The 'don't interrupt' rule (see page 15), can cause great problems. I have never really worked out how to say goodbye when leaving a group activity.

You can picture the scene – everyone standing round in twos & threes chatting, and I am going out. I'm not to interrupt anyone talking, and I wasn't with anyone in particular, so who do I say "goodbye" to? I've watched hundreds of others, over many years, who go out calling "goodbye" and others answer. I just can't work out what to do myself. I know that other people on the autistic spectrum have this problem, and some forget to try to say goodbye at all.

I also forget to invite people in if they come to my house. Well, it's not so much forget, as it never enters my head to do so. I suppose it's because visitors are so few and far between at my house. Naturally I ask social workers etc in, who come by appointment. A while ago, while a friend was visiting, I was providing respite care for a teenager at my home. His father came to collect him, and I answered the door and went to get the young man, so he could go home. My friend asked why I had left the father on the doorstep and not invited him in. I was amazed, the act hadn't occurred to me. My friend said I should have a sign by the door "if you know them, ask them in". Originally, I actually wrote a sign on a piece of card, but now it's just a mental sign, that reminds me when I answer the door. So if an autistic person doesn't invite you in, don't think they are being rude, it just hasn't occurred to them to do so.

IT WORKED FOR US!

Bryn repeatedly arrived home from his weekly after school club without his coat. The staff insisted he left the gym where the club was held with his coat, but lost it between there and the minibus outside.

This was unlikely as Bryn doesn't put down his belongings, so I suspected someone was taking it from him. After buying two expensive new winter coats in a month, I decided that something needed to be done.

I printed his initials as a monogram on some iron-on fabric with a picture of his favourite film character. My thoughts were that this would make the coat unattractive someone with different initials. He lost no more coats!

PROBLEM SOLVED !

(Iron-on printable fabric can be purchased from: www.craftycomputerpaper.co.uk)

B IS FOR BEING DIFFERENT

Do NT's (Neuro-Typical / non-autistics) feel like they are different people in different situations? I have always felt like I am at least two different people.

When I was younger, I felt a different person in school, at church & at home. It was even worse when I was away at college in South Wales, the train journey in between home & college, was when I changed 'beings'. I hated my Mum & Dad coming to college, as they were part of my 'other life', or when they came to church or Girls' Brigade, when I was younger. I was always eager to get rid of them, when they were in the 'wrong' place. In my day, parents weren't in school at the same time as children, parent's evenings were child-free zones, so there wasn't the same problem there.

When I was first diagnosed, I realised I felt different when I was with my family & their friends, to what I did the rest of the time. My extended family don't like me talking about having Asperger's Syndrome, so I have to behave differently with them, in an effort to be more like they want me to be, and don't feel quite like myself (i.e. how I am the rest of the time). It's not a conscious change of behaviour. My mind automatically changes tack, on the drive to my parent's house, or wherever we are meeting. I can be in floods of tears from my 'tunnels of hell' (see H is for Hell), but on the way out of the house, the 'Hell' stops. It immediately starts again when I leave them on my way home.

If my parents come into my work or social life, I have to be two people at once and generally try to keep my distance from them. In my own life, at my home, work, with friends, and with my children, I can be autistic and be myself.

My youngest son was at a residential special needs school. Like others in this situation, he learnt to do things at school e.g. wash hands/hang up clothes, but refused to do this at home. This is because the 'school Rhodri' did these things, but the 'home Rhodri' didn't. This wasn't much of a problem when he was in 52 week care and only home on Sundays. When he lived at home, or had longer holidays, this was difficult to cope with.

I remember when he had first started his day special school, at 3 years old, his teacher mentioned how he ate his meals with a fork, while at home he refused to do so and used his fingers. She suggested I visit the class to see him doing it. I called in to school one lunch time and, through the window in the door, watched the children settling down for lunch. Rhodri, with the others, then picked up his fork and started eating! The teacher came out and suggested I go into the class. I said to Rhodri "so you can use a fork then" and he looked guilty, showing he understood more than we thought!

Both my sons are more intelligent than they appear. Due to their lack of speech, both are taken for being unable to understand. Actually, they are both extremely intelligent in their own ways. Bryn is the fastest, most accurate typist that most people have ever seen. He uses all his fingers, as he learnt by watching me, and I learnt typewriting at college. He is now a lot faster than me! He spends most of his time on his computer, and normally requests new computer fonts for Christmas presents. These are often the only things on his list for Father Christmas, making it difficult when family ask what he would like for a present.

My 'different beings' are becoming more alike as I get older, and more confident, especially now I know I am different from most other people. I have managed to teach myself to join the world, although I often make mistakes and want to run away and hide.

I can also put on a 'professional front' and many times over the years have taught workshops and given talks to groups. Provided I have a good knowledge of my subject, I am able to do this without difficulty. It is the conversation with individuals after the group activity that I find the problem.

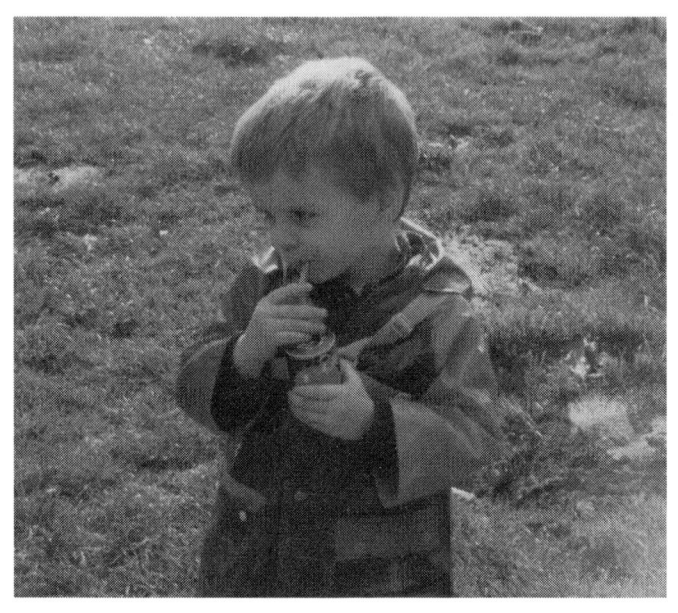

IT WORKED FOR US!

Rhodri grew out of a toddler sized harness and reins before he grew out of the need for them. I found that www.crelling.com sell harnesses and reins to fit up to adult size. They also sell harnesses for escapologists who refuse to keep their seat belts fastened in the car!

PROBLEM SOLVED !

C IS FOR CONVERSATION

I often used to say that neither of my children can talk. That was not strictly true, Bryn could actually speak words, but he didn't really use them for conversation. He could read any words (but not understand them), could repeat words & sentences from television programmes, understand some single words and could answer simple questions, yes or no. Bryn (now 23 years old) is starting to learn to speak sentences, to plan his day and explain what he wants to do, to those who support him. I had come to think that this would never come. Rhodri however, still can't say anything recognisable (at 21 years old), although he can vocalise a few sounds similar to those made by a baby.

As someone with Asperger's Syndrome, I have always had problems with initiating conversations. I think this was partly because of an occasion I remember from my junior school. I was in the fourth year (now called year 6). This was the year when I stopped 'talking'. I remember my teacher was Mr Bragg, the classroom was the first on the right in the school corridor, just past the girls' cloakroom. I remember sitting at a table near the window, and being in trouble <u>again</u>! I remember that I had said the wrong thing again – I'm not sure what it was. I think it may have been telling someone they had done something wrong. With my 'normal autistic' tendency to keep to rules, I tend to expect everyone else to keep to them too. I remember sitting and making a vow to myself that in future I would only answer questions from the teacher (or others in authority) and otherwise not talk, and that I would do exactly what I was told. I began to sit in silence, keeping my head down and letting the talk from teacher and children go over my head. This was useful on the day a few years later, when one teacher threw a wooden blackboard eraser at a pupil, which literally went over my head! (in 1973) I spoke to teachers, and to other people, when I really had to do so, as I knew I would be punished if I didn't.

As an adult, I started to realise I couldn't 'talk' when I was going to antenatal classes, when I was expecting Bryn. Everyone sat round in a circle, no-one knew anyone else, as usually you don't get pregnant at the same time as a friend! As I looked round, everyone (except me) was talking, laughing etc. and I was sat in silence on my own. I was madly trying to think of something to say to someone.

I have always been told that I was shy, and could talk if I tried – however I realised I wasn't actually shy, I desperately wanted to talk to someone, but there were no words in my mind. I decided I would have to find some words for the following weeks. So, when friends of my parents asked me questions e.g. "do you want a boy or a girl?", "when are you due?" etc. I committed the questions to memory. This gave me something to say to someone at my next class.

I really went on from there, learning sentences and questions that I could use when required. I spend a lot of time talking to myself in my mind. I used to work out pretend conversations on subjects (often autism/aspergers – my specialist subject!). In this way I built up a bank of 'sentences'. Fortunately I managed to adjust the 'sentences' slightly if required, and didn't always need new ones. If I knew I was going to have a discussion with someone, I would practice the conversation in my mind over the day or two (or more!) before. I was able to work out alternative 'sentences' depending on whether the other person says, yes or no, to questions of mine.

Sometimes someone would ask me something that I haven't answered before or I would be in a situation that hadn't occurred before, and I needed to say something. In these cases, I would sometimes go 'blank' and would, again, have no words to say. On these occasions, I had to change the subject, with another prearranged sentence, or mutter something and wander off. It's like walking into a 'room' for that subject and finding it empty - I search all the cupboards in the 'room' but nothing's there – I have to leave that 'room' and find another one. Later, when on my own, I rehearsed that question until I found an answer, which I could 'save' in case the subject came up again. I don't normally need to do this now, as my communication has improved tremendously. However, if I am in 'autistic mode' due to extreme stress, this 'empty head syndrome' as I always think of it, can return and once more, I am lost for words.

If children don't know what to say to make friends, it would help if they learnt 'sentences' which are suitable as conversation starters, as I did. As an adult, I learnt suitable sentences from other adults. I have known parents trying to teach their children what to say. It is often of little help to them if, for example, a 10 yr old starts talking in the language of a 40 yr old in the playground! The youngsters need to learn from someone nearer their own age – a friendly, helpful teenager perhaps? Preferably of the same sex as them.

I also have problems when I get lost in a conversation and forget what I'm saying, particularly if interrupted. I seem to be getting worse with this lately, and wonder if it's now due to old age setting in! I can't always keep up with what people are saying and my mind wanders. I went to meetings e.g. at the Care Forum, for months, before I was able to learn the 'language', and to contribute, and even now, I'm often 'lost' about what people are talking about.

When I ran a parent support group, I could organise the room, the refreshments, newsletters etc, but I had to ask someone else to come to lead the conversation. Particularly if there were going to be parents without autistic children, so I was unable to talk about my specialist subject!

I'm generally better with written language, than spoken language, and don't have the same problems with writing letters etc, and prefer email to telephone conversations.

When Rhodri was about 6 or 7 years old, I became very frustrated at his lack of communication. I had known for some time that he could read – he could distinguish between the many video tapes with ease, and could point to words like toilet when we were out. I read on the internet, of a communication system called PECS (Picture Exchange Communication System). There were examples of cards with a drawing and a word, for everyday objects. It was possible download these to print out, and I did so, but as it was an American website, a lot of the words were wrong. As I knew that Rhodri could read some words, I printed out my own cards with just the words on them. I attached magnets to the cards, and put them on a large magnetic board on the wall in the hall.

I remember the first time I introduced them to Rhodri. I had started with about six words on the board. The first one was BATH. I picked it off the board, showed it to Rhodri and told him the name, then went to the bath and pointed saying "Bath". That evening, I picked up the card, showed him, and he gave me a big smile and went immediately into the bathroom and started getting undressed. He hadn't done this on his own before. I followed up with more words. I can't remember them all now, but they were things like DINNER, BED, TEA, DRINK, CAKE…..

As this had been a success, I decided that words to take out of the house would be a good idea. These would help me to tell Rhodri where we were going, and enable him to be able to make a choice. I therefore made cards saying GRANDMA'S, SAINSBURYS, PARK …. Along with cards for things we might need when out e.g. TOILET, DRINK… For these, I put a hole in the cards and attached them to a ring. With a cord attached, I could clip this on my belt and give the cards to Rhodri to choose what he wanted. He could also reach them, if he would like to initiate conversation. There were about 15 cards on the ring, some of which had different words on both sides.

This was very successful and the Social Work Assistant, who came regularly to take Rhodri out, said that she was proud for her name to be on one of Rhodri's cards. I had added a card with her name, so I could point to it when we were waiting for her to arrive so he could go out.

Later, Rhodri's school at the time, decided to start using PECS and insisted he start at the beginning, using the cards with pictures and no words. He wasn't very good at this, and it was a shame that despite my insistence they wouldn't let him use the words. Fortunately as a teenager, he was given a word book, which is what he still uses. He carries it around with him, pointing to what he wants to say.

However having no speech, and his 'words' in his book being mainly restricted to nouns e.g. toilet, biscuit, drink .. there is no way for Rhodri to say what he really thinks. We can guess if he likes some places or activities by his behaviour at them, but that is all.

Bryn on the other hand, is better able to indicate his likes and dislikes, even if only using the words "Yes OK" and "No". He never says "yes" on its own, only "Yes OK" These answers are not always helpful as, although "No" means No, "Yes OK" can mean several things. It can mean Yes, but it equally can mean "I don't understand the question" or " I want you to go away".

When I founded a charity for disabled children, I used to produce regular newsletters. Although I always asked for articles to be send by email, so I could 'copy and paste' into the newsletter, someone gave me a long printed article. It was interesting, but amounted to two A4 pages of typing in reasonably small print. I thought "it will take me ages to type that in", then it occurred to me to ask Bryn if he would do it – he is a faster and more accurate typist than me. I took it and asked him, and he immediately opened a word document and started typing. I stayed to watch, as I wanted the resulting document saved to a file. Left on his own, he may have just closed it after he finished typing – because it wasn't something he would want to save. However, the plan didn't work. Bryn rapidly typed until he got to the middle of the second paragraph where the first mention of the word 'Autism' was – he immediately stopped said "No", gave it to me, and went back to what he was doing when I came in.

I have noticed also, that he gets very upset when the words 'Autism' or 'Autistic' are mentioned in his hearing. Originally, I thought this was due him not liking to be talked about, but it happens even if he is not the subject of conversation. I assume from this that he doesn't like being autistic, but will have to wait for his communication to improve further before he is in a position to tell me.

As for myself, although I sometimes hate having Asperger's Syndrome, and the various social problems, it is 'normal' for me – and I often think I wouldn't be me if I didn't have it. If only people would see my good points. I like to be nice to others, and try to help anyone when I can, and not upset them, but I often seem to be permanently in trouble for doing the wrong thing.

Sometimes Brynmor's speech pattern deteriorates into what it was in the past. He has always had echolalia, i.e. he repeats the last thing he hears. This does not happen so much these days, but if he is feeling 'off' for some reason, he answers questions by repeating the end of the question. For example: Asking him "What do you want in your sandwich? Cheese or Ham?" would receive the response "Ham".

I can sometimes tell if he is answering or just being echolalic, as if he gives a 'real' answer, he will take a short time to think of the answer. An echolalic reply will come immediately. If I'm not sure, I may then test him by asking "Do you want Ham or Cheese?" and if he says "Cheese", I know not to trust either answer as he won't actually be indicating a choice, simply repeating what I'm saying. In this case I'd give him cheese, as he rarely eats ham!

It was due to echolalia, that when he started at residential college, he spent the first few months living on Cheese Salad. The main meal of the day was taken in the college restaurant at mid-day. The college contacted me after he had been there a few weeks, to say that they were concerned that he only had cheese salad every day for lunch, and the evening meal was only a snack.

Having discussed the issue with them, it turned out that the menu always had 'cheese salad' as the last thing. So when it was read to him, he always replied with this. I suggested they tell him the meals on offer in a different order, but by then the cheese salad was not only because it was the last thing, but was a routine, so he continued to request nothing else. I told them to stop asking him for a week or two, and to give him something else without asking him what he wanted. I suggested to them some meals that he liked. This worked, and soon they were able to ask him, without him insisting on cheese salad all the time.

This wasn't the first time that this sort of thing happened. He had pizza for lunch every day at junior school for years, as it was the last thing on the menu – and he doesn't even like pizza! The staff were unhelpful when I suggested that pizza every day wasn't a balanced diet. Matters were solved when he went onto a gluten free diet, as there was often only one gluten free item on the menu, and it wasn't pizza! (see page 111). It did annoy me that they insisted he chose his meal from the list every day, with the other children, then told him he couldn't have his choice as "Mum says you can't have that, you have to have (the gluten free option)".

IT WORKED FOR US!

Bryn had problems remembering to wear clean underwear each day. He was able to remember to change his socks, as we bought them showing the days of the week. I printed the days of the week on some printable iron-on material and ironed them on each pair of pants. I made two for each day, as otherwise if one was in the wash he wouldn't wear any at all!

I also found it helpful to make name labels with my sons' photographs and telephone number, to help lost clothes come home! One teacher used to look in Rhodri's coat for my number if he wanted to phone me, he said it was quicker than looking on the computer!

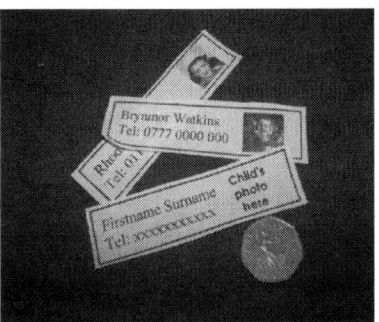

PROBLEM SOLVED !

D IS FOR DAYDREAMS

I can't remember when I first had a 'dream world'. They varied over the years, but the common factor was that in my 'dream worlds' people liked me, and I had lots of friends. This was a complete contrast to my real world.

The first imaginary 'friend' I can remember, was an imaginary dog. I used to walk home from junior school 'with' him, as I was lonely being on my own. His name was Bounce – named after a dog food sold in my Grandpa's shop. I never told anyone about him, as I knew other people, like my mum, would tell me not to be silly. By the time I was in secondary school, I had a 'dream world', that I was able to 'escape' into at any time.

I continued to 'escape' into those other worlds for most of my life. I could do things in the 'real world' e.g. go for a walk, do the housework, go shopping etc. when my mind was not wholly there. I had to make myself give up my 'dream worlds' when I was responsible for Brynmor & Rhodri. They both needed 1:1 continuous care, and I couldn't do this if my mind kept wandering.

In later years, I wished I was able to 'escape' as completely as I used to, but I have now lost the ability, and the 'worlds'. My mind now continually rehearses conversations and situations based on activities throughout the day and expectations of future occurrences. I sometime 'escape' into thinking what to

write for this book. I go over and over words in my brain. The other way I 'escape' is using the computer.
I play a game like solitaire or bookworm (finding words in a grid) over and over, to stop my mind 'exploding' and calm me down. I also use the computer most of the evening, entering competitions, or reading craft forums. I can't just watch TV and not do anything else.

I can still 'lose' myself in a book. Mostly I read detective stories, which need to be puzzled out. I sometimes read myself to sleep, to stop my mind tormenting itself on other matters. I'm particularly keen on audio books, but mostly those stories when I already have the written books/videos. Listening to audio books while doing housework/cooking/gardening etc. also stops my mind going haywire. As I know the story anyway, it doesn't matter if I miss a bit of the narrative while working.

I have found that meditation can be very relaxing, but it took a long time for me to get the hang of it. I have learnt to do Reiki, and can use it to heal myself and other people, this has helped to relax me. Reiki is a simple Japanese energy-balancing method that is used by hundreds of people all over the world. Reiki helps me to think positively, and to mostly keep the autistic part of my brain away. Otherwise, when I am getting stressed, I can feel the autism coming into my brain and I begin to panic. I understand, by talking to others, that I do not normally show I am worried and anxious, having become expert at hiding my emotions, so no-one else knows it is happening.

E IS FOR EYE CONTACT

Before I started this book, I went to a course about teaching social skills to children with autism. I have difficulty with this, due to not knowing the skills myself. I always find these sorts of talks very odd. It's all "people with autism do this, while as you know, we all do that". I'm then left thinking "oh, that's what you do is it?" It's by going to these talks that I can find out how non-autistic people normally think, and sometimes am surprised that they have to be told things obvious to me. It was due to this, I decided to write some articles which turned into this book.

There was a lot of discussion about Eye Contact. I didn't actually find out what eye contact was, until I was diagnosed with Autism/Asperger's Syndrome aged 40. For years before that, teachers, doctors etc, kept saying (about my sons) "They haven't got eye contact, have they?" Well, with several people in a meeting saying that, I wasn't about to disagree, although I was always thinking "There's nothing wrong with their eyes". I just agreed to keep them happy. Later, when I found out what it was, I realised I hadn't noticed, as I didn't have it either!

When I went to my GP, to say I thought I was Autistic, and could she refer me to my sons' psychiatrist, she asked me if I did anything 'odd'. I said it was difficult to answer that, as I obviously didn't think myself 'odd'. One thing I could tell her about, which I knew was odd, (because my husband used to laugh at me) was when I had a bath, I turned all the children's ducks, so they weren't looking at me.

Another thing that helped me find out about eye contact, was that I became friendly with someone who is deaf and who lip-reads. I was told "If you want to talk to 'Anne', you have to look at her". But I couldn't – looking at someone's face made me feel sick. Luckily, I realised that I had been told wrong – I only had to have my mouth facing her, I could be looking anywhere, so normally I actually looked over her shoulder. After a few months, as I got used to this, I got to thinking "this is **** stupid, what can 'Anne' do to me, if I look at her". I asked her if I could practice looking at her, but I had to physically hold her hand (for comfort) to be able to do so. When I got used to it, I stopped holding hands, and can now usually look at other people when I talk to them too. When having a stressful conversation, I can feel my autism taking over and realise that I am losing eye contact with the other person.

This also brings back a memory of the first appointment I had for Bryn (then aged 3 and a half) to see the community paediatrician at his nursery school. Bryn was lining up blocks on her desk. Rhodri was in my arms, as he was a baby. I was looking down at Rhodri, but he started staring at my face, and I shuddered and looked away. The doctor noticed and said, "Are you alright?" I told her I hated it when he did that, because it made me feel sick. She said, "that's interesting", and asked if Bryn had also done that. I said "no", and she said that was because Bryn was autistic and Rhodri wasn't. Actually, as it turns out now, Rhodri is more autistic that Bryn – he lost his staring at faces by the time he was 2 years old.

If I don't look at faces, I normally try to find something on the person to concentrate on, whether it's a tie, badge or pattern on a shirt etc. It means I'm looking the right way, but just not at their face.

There is not much point in asking an autistic person to look at your face, when you are talking to them. No one can concentrate on listening, when feeling sick, or in pain, although I do ask my sons to look in my direction, and not face the other way. I think it would help if teachers etc wore a coloured badge, and pointed and said, "look at that, when I'm talking to you", then they could be sure that the person was paying attention, rather than insist on eye contact.

I feel scared when approached by people wearing dark sunglasses. I mean those that look black, the lighter brown/shaded ones are less threatening, which is fortunate as Bryn wears these. The completely black glasses look like large eyes looking at me.

Similarly I used to hate it when my Mum would point out an inanimate object, e.g. a house with windows & door which were in the right positions to be eyes, nose & mouth. She would say "Oh look, that looks like a face looking at you!", and tell me not to be so silly when I said I didn't want to look at it, as it scared me.

IT WORKED FOR US!

Rhodri sometimes pinches the driver in a car. Often this is because he is trying to say something, but it could cause an accident. We now have clear acrylic screens which can be fixed to the back of the front seats. He is enclosed in the back, and unable to reach to touch the driver or front passenger.

PROBLEM SOLVED !

http://safeshield-ltd.co.uk will give a donation to "The Brandon Trust" who provide work training for people with learning difficulties (including Bryn) for all orders resulting from being mentioned in this book.

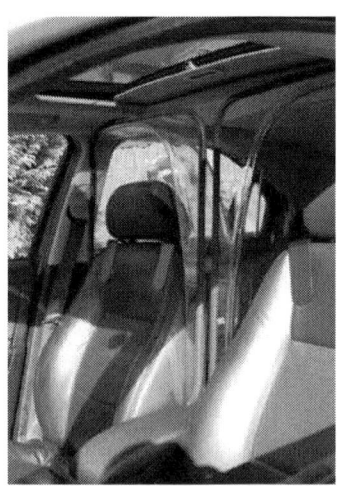

F IS FOR FRIENDS

They say that people with Autism don't see the need for friends, and people with Asperger's want friends and don't know how to get them.

What is a friend? According to the dictionary it's "a person whom you know well and whom you like a lot, but who is usually not a member of your family."

In infant school, I can't remember having a friend. My mum tells me, I was sorry for the little boy I sat next to, as he kept getting told off.

In junior school, I took ages (from Sept until about April) to make a friend – the school had the policy to mix the three classes for the following year, and to separate friends – so I had to start again next September. Between the 3rd & 4th years (now called yr. 5 & 6), someone must have noticed my problem and I was put in to same class as my friend from the 3rd year. I managed to make another friend, as well, having two friends was a big achievement!

Neither of my junior school friends went to the same secondary school as me. In fact only one person in my class went there – one I didn't like, naturally. I made a friend in the first year. We didn't have much in common, but she was a kindly girl and, I think, she was sorry for me being on my own. The following September, she stopped to talk to a girl with spina bifida and what is now termed 'learning difficulties', in the corridor, who she knew from Junior School. Her name was Angela and was in the year below us, she asked if my friend would like to play cards with her at lunchtime, as she had to stay in the classroom. My friend said "no", but I said I would and I did so, and remained friendly with Angela until she died aged 26.

This was a 'godsend' for me, as I didn't have to socialise in the playground at break times and lunchtimes. I only saw my class in lesson times. I often think that this is how I survived school! I was usually safe in lesson times as teachers had more control of the classes in those days – it was outside class that there were the problems with bullying etc.

In the first year of the sixth form, I met up again with one of my junior school friends, who had transferred schools to retake 'O levels'. I wasn't able to see Angela at school, as the sixth form was separate. Angela later moved to a residential special needs college and I didn't see her much afterwards, we drifted apart as I was away at college or working and had less time.

I was mostly on my own at college, taking an HND in Mathematics, Statistics and Computing, and spent a lot of time in the library. I met my future husband at college, he was the only person in my class who really spoke to me.

At several evening classes, other people have been friendly – sometimes only because they could borrow my cake decorating equipment – I always leant things, in an attempt to be nice to people. Several times however, I discovered that when I didn't have a particular cutter, and asked to borrow one, they refused. It seemed borrowing only went one way!

I partly got married in order to leave home, as I was finding my parents too difficult to live with permanently, especially after being away at college. In 1996, after being married ten years, we separated, although we aren't actually divorced, as neither of us has a new partner.

As an adult, I have always found difficulty in finding friends. I generally had people who were friendly in several of my work situations or other organisations, but no-one to meet with outside. When I finally managed to find a 'friend' who I met through a carer's group, my children would not let her come to my house, if they were in. The eldest would say "Goodbye, goodbye" and try to push her out. She said my children were 'bad' and wanted me to themselves. I tried to explain it was because they had never experienced visitors before. Other people (social workers etc) who came to visit, always did so in school time. The only visitors I had were those who were paid to be there. As my children had spent all their lives with just Mum (& originally Dad) at home, they didn't understand the concept of visitors. They will accept people coming in if I went out, e.g. babysitters, but not if I am there as well.

How do you know if someone is a friend? I don't know.
I have discovered that it is not enough for them to say "I'm your friend" as they may be lying. Experience has

shown me that someone who says "I will be your friend forever" is normally the first to reject you.

Can friendships be one way? If you like someone, and would like them as a friend, but they don't like you in the same way, perhaps they are sorry for you, or think you need help, and you can be their 'good deed'. Unfortunately people get tired of 'good deeds' and move on to the next – leaving the 'friend' behind, wondering what has happened and feeling hurt.

Several 'friends' have told me they only became friendly with me because another friend of theirs told them to do so. It was noticed I was always on my own, so this 'friend' invited me to visit them. They encouraged me to phone/email them if I would like to visit them for a chat and a cup of tea. However, I always discover that this is a 'one-way' friendship. The 'friend' never suggests to me that we meet.

After several years of this with one 'friend', when I visited her once a week or two, I decided that I was fed up with a one-sided friendship – she refused to come to my house, saying she didn't need to as I could come to her. So I stopped contacting her, deciding to wait to see if she missed me and how long it would take for her to make contact with me. <u>Eighteen months</u> later, I received a Christmas Card – She hadn't missed me much!

My 'friends' often prove to only want me because I can provide something, normally a lift in my car. I never know if I'm actually liked, or just tolerated as a means to an end. Years ago, I had a 'friend' who I met through one of my sons' schools. She asked me if I would like to go to a craft group with her, that she hadn't been to before, then she told me I would have to pick her up in the car as her husband needed theirs. She used to ask me round her house for a cup of tea sometimes, and I thought I had found a friend at last.

I wasn't keen on the craft group, the other members being well-off and looked down at me for not having the latest equipment etc. So when my mum wanted me to go to a meeting with her on the same night of the month, I was glad of the excuse and apologised to my 'friend' saying my mum needed a lift. 'Friend' said not to worry, 'Mavis' had said she lived near and could give her a lift anytime I couldn't go – and that was the last I heard of her! I tried a couple of phone messages, Christmas card etc, saying about meeting for a cuppa, but heard nothing from her again!

Now Bryn has finished college, and is living at home, it is difficult not being able to have anyone come to the house. I can only invite people here at very limited times when he is out. He sometimes accepts visitors if he is told when the person is leaving. He says "Going home at?" It is best for me to overestimate the stay to give a time, or the visitor will be shown he/she is very unwelcome at the allotted time, if he/she is still here. This has happened to several social workers, one of whom seemed not to understand what "goodbye, goodbye" screamed in her face actually meant, as she asked if he wanted her to leave! I have several times had to finish interviewing potential support workers in the front garden, as continuing to talk in the house was impossible.

If anyone with Asperger's Syndrome is reading this chapter in the hope of finding out how to make friends, then I have to say I don't have an answer. I think it is easier to resign myself to being on my own. Joining groups where someone may talk to me occasionally, gives a pretence that I have friends. I have had 'paid friends' in some of Bryn's support workers and, once a social worker, however it's necessary to always remember that these people will at some point change their jobs and leave.

At one time I was being considered for a job supporting a young man with Asperger's Syndrome. The person telling me about the job, mentioned that the young man wanted to know how to make friends – I decided not to go for the position, as I knew I would be no help there at all.

Having just found myself on my own again, having been 'dumped' by two 'friends', I'm looking for a new group to join. About 15 years ago, I used to do craft demonstrations and workshops for women's groups, and I am starting to do this again – in an effort to make some friends or at least find some company. I also plan to give some talks about autism, based on this book.

G IS FOR GROWING UP

Becoming an adult is difficult for autistic young people, partly because their interests remain the same as when they were children. Bryn & Rhodri (now in their twenties) both still love watching Thomas the Tank Engine. Yet, when Bryn started his special needs secondary school at 11 yrs old, I was told by the teacher to replace the lunch box he had chosen, which had Thomas on it, as it was not age-appropriate.

It's also difficult for parents to come to terms with their children getting older and going to college or moving into residential care. When you have had to do everything for your child for 20+ years, it's even more difficult to 'let go' than for most other parents.

Over the years, I have supported adults with learning difficulties in various situations and have realised that many people have trouble with not behaving as if the older adults concerned are children. I have known people with learning difficulties, in their 40's who are told they are "naughty". Grown men are told "good boy" when they do something well! How inappropriate is that remark! I was told by one such adult that I hadn't said "good boy", I replied that I wouldn't say that as he wasn't a child or a dog. He gave me a big smile, as he hated being treated as a child. My youngest son's residential home says "good man". I hate this remark as well. Who says "good man" in the outside world? When I do something well, e.g. icing a cake that someone likes, they said "well done", "that's good", "that's great Lynne" or something similar not "good woman"! I would have thought it would be better to say "Good (name)" saying the person's name.

On a similar line, I had an issue with Bryn's teacher who complained at a review meeting, that they had difficulty getting him to shake hands. It was explained he was supposed to shake hands and say "Good morning" to the teacher and each of the members of his class every morning. I asked "why?" and the teacher said it was to teach them to be polite. I said "so every morning when you go into the staff room, you shake hands with all the other teachers and say 'good morning'?" He said "well, no". So, I asked, why teach the children such out-dated behaviour. Shaking hands with everyone all the time, hasn't been the norm for over 50 years. I sometimes shake hands with strangers on our first meeting, but not those I know well. I pointed out he hadn't shook my hand when we met that afternoon. I really hate it when autistic children (and adults) are taught behaviour that will make them stand out as 'different' when they have enough differences without these extras.

Another problem with supporting adults is to remember that they should have some control over their own lives, and should not be 'told what to do' or to be reprimanded like speaking to a child. I try to advise rather than give instructions and say things like "If I were you ....." or "It might be better if ......" I find this method is appreciated by the adult concerned and leads to less conflicting behaviour and anxiety.

H IS FOR HELL

I'm always thinking of 'something'. I can't think of 'nothing'. My mind is often busy with two or three layers of thoughts at the same time. Always at the back of my mind is the layer of thought that repeats images and/or sentences. Sometimes I hate being autistic, I hate my mind that won't switch off, I hate the sentences (see below), I just hate being me, I just want to die.

I recently came to know my spirit guide (you might say guardian angel), who says she has been with me since I was born. It's a wonder she stuck with me that long – 50 years of going from one disaster to the next.

I have just had another 'disaster', where my life has fallen apart. Due to a lack of friends and social situations, I tend to only have one at a time. I then become too reliant on the situation/friend, and am unable to cope if the connection is cut.

Actually, I was in the unusual position (for me) of having two friends at the time. This has happened before, when I was in the sixth form, I had a friend from school and one at church. Not Angela mentioned before, as she was away at her special needs college at the time. One weekend, shortly after we had left school, the school friend stayed Saturday night at my home, after accompanying me to a family party as there were no-one else my age attending. The next morning, my mother asked if I was going to church & I said I wasn't as my school friend was there, and she didn't attend church. My Mum said I should take her, and introduce her to my 'church friend'. As someone who always did as she was told, I did so. 'School friend' found she enjoyed the church service, she came again to the evening service and to the youth meeting afterwards, and started attending each week.

About a month later, I was told by a third party, that 'school friend' and 'church friend' were going shopping & to the cinema together. Neither had ever suggested anything like this to me, I only met them at each of our houses, school or church. I had never been anywhere else with either of them. Then they went off to sit together in church each week, where there were only two available seats, and I was left alone sitting at the back and in a corner at the youth meeting.

I had fallen foul of the 'trap' of introducing two 'friends' to each other and finding they preferred each other to me. This happened again about 15 years ago, and again recently. I never seem to learn – I'm always trying to be nice by taking one person to another place I go to, but I end up alone and pushed out.

My 'tunnels of hell' revolve around the fact that my mind is repetitive. I think that is the best way to describe it. In my 'D is for Daydreams' chapter, I wrote "My mind now continually rehearses conversations and situations based on activities throughout the day and expectations of future occurrences". While in a 'tunnel of hell', I get my 'sentences' as I call them. These are repetitions of what people have said to me. The usual way that 'friends' get rid of me is to say; "You are taking up too much of my time", "You don't deserve friends", then there are other 'sentences' about me being a bad person etc.

So, when 'dumped' by a 'friend', my mind just repeats over and over, whatever 'put down' sentences she has come up with, to torture me. Then all the other 'sentences' from previous 'friends' (and others) come back too. This means that every time I'm in this situation, I get more 'sentences of torture'. Twenty four hours a day, except during my three or four hours of sleep a night (having taken melatonin), the 'sentences' repeat themselves – shouting over and over in my brain. The only way I have found to stop them is to play my ipod at top volume into my head with earphones. My ipod is now my lifeline, I'm never without it.

I call this a 'tunnel of hell'. The 'sentences' normally stay in a cupboard in my mind, and at the time of writing, I have managed to put them all back. I'm still left with the accompanying panic, and worries about the future, fears of doing the wrong thing and of everyone hating me.

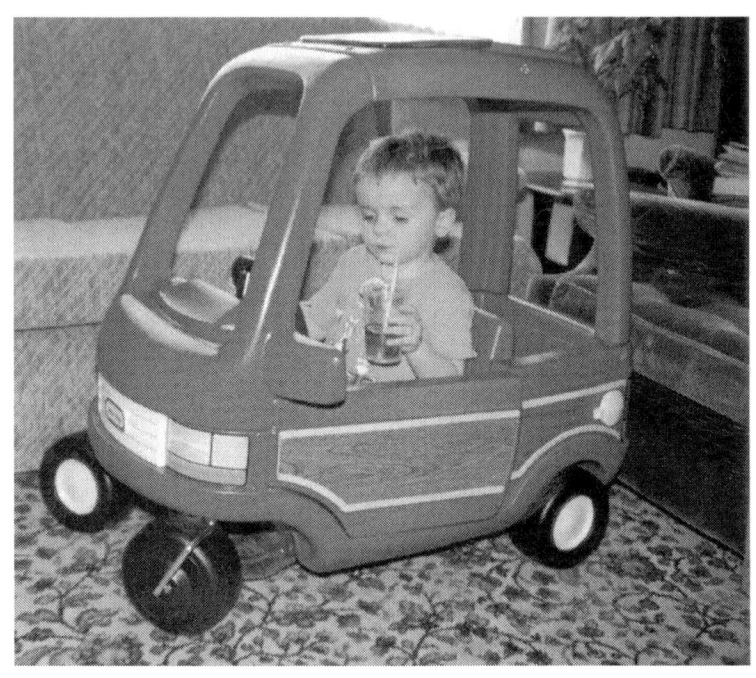

In 1994, Rhodri loved the 'Little Tykes' car he received for his third birthday. Unfortunately, he also loved climbing on the roof, so he could go over the fence into next door's garden!

I is for Imagination

A while ago, I went to an afternoon event for carers, i.e. people who care for a disabled person without pay (normally a family member). The event included an afternoon tea and activities at a local community centre. The workshops on offer were "Singing", "Paper crafts" and "Fun with Words". Everyone had to sign up for one session.

I was stuck for which would be best to do. I was uncomfortable being at the event in the first place and had wondered whether to stay at home, as I had to go on my own. I persuaded myself to attend as I was trying to advertise my Reiki treatments and had some leaflets to give to the organisation holding the event, as I wished to offer half price treatments to carers.

So, I was left with choosing a workshop. "Singing" was definitely out – I am tone deaf, and my singing is generally likened to moaning by other people hearing me. "Paper crafts" was quite appealing, as I am very good at crafts, having been 'making things' since a young child. However, I knew from previous such events that there was a problem with me taking this workshop i.e. I was likely to be better than everyone else… As someone who has taught workshops and who demonstrates crafts for groups, I would probably end up giving help to others. While this would not be a problem and I would be happy to do this, I know from experience that other teachers can resent this, and I hate 'standing out' when people say "why is yours, better than mine..?".

So, as I was already uncomfortable being at the event, I opted for "Fun with Words", to hopefully solve my problem. I vaguely thought that this meant something like crossword puzzles, but unfortunately it was "Creative Writing". Ah well, I thought, it might help with this book. It has, but only by being a subject for this chapter.

The workshop tutor started by asking us to "pretend you are a biscuit, what biscuit would you be and why?" What? I'm not a biscuit? How can I pretend I'm a biscuit?? I was a blank, while others decided to be custard creams or other types of biscuits. Then we were asked to choose a famous person and describe what article of furniture they could be and why... At this point, I switched off. While others were writing about their article of furniture, I started my chapter on "I is for imagination – lack of!"

I have never been very good at imagination. At school, when we had to write an essay in English Language, I always chose the factual option, rather than one of the fictional essays. Once I remember, when asked to write a story about how the world began, I wrote the story as it happened in the bible and was told that was wrong. Apparently, I was supposed to invent what had happened. I couldn't understand what I was supposed to write, as I believed the bible story about how the world began and had therefore, I considered, written the truth.

J IS FOR JULY

"July", I hear you say, "What has July to do with Autism?"

Well nothing – but is my birthday month, and that brings me onto birthday (& other) parties.

I have always hated parties, and not wanted one. When I was young, children of friends of my mother, started being friendly to me at the end of June each year – Obviously having been told by their mums "Be nice to Lynne and she will ask you to her party" – they ignored or taunted me the rest of the year. My Mum decided whom I was asking to my party, and asked them, so they thought they had got away with it, and I didn't know.

I remember the last year in Junior School (now called year 6) when I managed to convince my Mum that now I was going to be 11 years old, I was too old for parties. I was also terrified that year, because 'the bumps' had just become popular for birthdays, when children held your arms and legs and bumped you up and down on the ground, for the number of years of your birthday. I was petrified of letting anyone know the exact date of my birthday. I managed to get away with only asking one girl to tea, and didn't tell her it was my birthday, until we were on the way home from school. I had learnt that 'the bumps' had to be on the exact day, so the following day was too late for them to get me.

I didn't have a party again until I was 18 and leaving the 6th form, when I did have a group of 4 friends, to ask to my house. That is the largest amount of friends, I have ever had at one time. We were all 'misfits' in the 6th form, who met up at break & lunchtimes. However none of them stayed in contact after we left school.

I can't say I like birthdays now, they just seem like other days, except I get a present and a card from my parents. One year, I received 6 cards – a big achievement! Another year, I didn't get any cards, as my Mum & Dad were on holiday. My children don't understand birthdays and having presents, because they have never had anyone to ask to a party either. They used to take a birthday cake to school or activity club, so everyone could sing "Happy Birthday" and they could blow out the candles, but now birthdays are 'normal days' for them too, except for presents from myself & their grandparents.

I still hate parties, but very rarely get asked to one anyway. I can't walk into a crowded room by myself, without knowing where I'm going to sit. So for parties, meetings etc, I always get there early. I find a seat, near the door and on the end of a row, or possibly in a corner and put my coat on it. Then I have my 'base' if I need to leave the room for the toilet etc. I can go back to my 'base' and sit down. I'm not so bad if I am with someone, but unless I'm with my Mum, I'm usually on my own.

K IS FOR KEEP HOPING

"Everything comes to those who wait!"

Bryn (then aged 17) had a cold and had just taken some tablets (paracetamol and echinacea) for it. He had always refused any medicine (liquid or tablets) from as soon as he had been able to 'fight back'. Even as a young child, I was unable to get any medicines into him. If he was so ill with an infection that he was 'floppy', I was usually able to lie on him to hold his legs down, hold his arms with one hand and squeeze some liquid medicine into his mouth with an oral syringe with the other hand. After about 2 days, he would have recovered too much for this to work, as he was very strong.

I tried 'putting it into a drink', but he could taste it and then refused all drinks, in case I tried to trick him again, which is not helpful if someone is ill and needs to drink a lot of liquid. At one time, there was a strawberry flavour antibiotic that hid reasonably well in milkshake, but then our usual chemist changed their supplier and had orange flavour which was hopeless. I had to go round all the local chemists, asking what flavour their antibiotics were, before handing in the prescription! The chemists never seemed to understand my problems, and I sometimes received a different flavour to the one they had originally said they would give me. The milkshake method only worked for a couple of days too, before Bryn discovered what I was doing.

I then hit on the idea of asking the GP for a stronger medicine, so he would need less of it. Then, if I got it in his mouth, when he spat it out a greater concentration would stay around his mouth and would be swallowed with a drink. We were prescribed one that he only had to take half a teaspoon, using an oral syringe, which worked for a few days. Bryn has never finished a course of antibiotics, as one is always told to do, but he is now a very healthy person, rarely even getting a cold!

When he was about 16 years old, I discovered some painkillers that could dissolve in the mouth without needing to be swallowed – naturally these tasted better than usual. When he had a headache, I broke them into small pieces and fed them to Bryn with a drink of water afterwards. This was a success and when he was ill, the GP gave me a prescription for them as they are expensive if you need a lot. He will now take Omega-3, zinc & vitamin capsules by dropping them in a glass of water and drinking them, and will take ordinary paracetamols by putting them straight in his mouth.

Everything comes to those who wait!

I often thought when my sons were small, is there ever an end to this? Will this ever get better?

I remember taking Bryn to buy shoes – another 'sit on him' activity – child screaming, kicking, hanging upside down over my lap… Those of you with autistic children will know what I mean, I'm sure.

One day we went into the shoe shop and Bryn sat and tried on shoes – reasonably quietly. They were OK, so we went to pay. The shop assistant said "That's not the same child you had last time is it?" It was! By now, I couldn't get Rhodri into the shop at all, and had to buy him 'the next size up' from a shop where they didn't insist children try on shoes, and let you return any that didn't prove to fit. However, from aged 15, Rhodri was able to try on shoes in a shop, but he takes them off again quickly. Starting Rhodri wearing new shoes, generally involves hiding his old ones. So either he goes out with new shoes, or stays in. This means he puts his new shoes on, as he wants to go out.

Haircuts used to be similar problem. I initially tried taking Bryn (aged about 3) to the hairdresser, but they refused to cut the hair of a wriggling child. When he started at his first special school, the teacher asked if I would like her to cut his hair. She used to bring some electric clippers, line the children up watching a video, and cut the hair of those whose parents wished her to do so, which was most of them!. As the children could see each other having their hair cut, and they were used to doing what they were told at school, they all went home looking tidy. It was fortunate for me as at that time, both my sons were in the same class! When Bryn left the school to move to an autistic unit attached to a mainstream school, I had to buy my own clippers! I still cut his hair now, as he insists on stripping to his underpants when this happens. I think he doesn't like any bits of hair on his clothes.

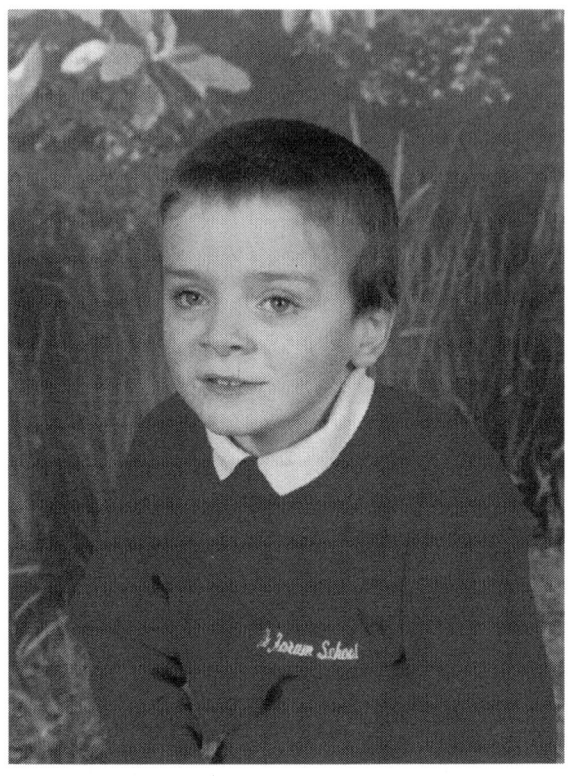

Rhodri was very happy at the Forum School, he loved wearing his uniform sweatshirt. See page 90

L is for Letters

My Mum was recently telling me that I weighed just over 5lb when I was born, and just escaped spending time in an incubator, due to being able to breathe by myself. I was obviously born a fighter! I have continued all my life to fight. I often have to fight myself.

I have things I'm unable to do, because of my autism. I am unable to go to places on my own for the first time. Even I know that this is completely illogical, but it is something I can't do. If I go shopping, I will visit the large stores e.g. WHSmith, Sainsburys, Marks & Spencer which are basically the same everywhere, but going into independent shops which are unique to that place is difficult. I will 'eye them up' from outside for a while. If there is a large window area, giving a good view of the inside of the shop, then I may go in, but if I can't see what is in there, I won't. I can't go into a café/pub/restaurant on my own, even if I have been in there before. I have never been able to do this. I remember often whenever I was on holiday with my Mum & Dad and my children. When we were looking for a place for lunch, we would drive up to a pub, and need to look at the menu to see if they served anything gluten-free. My Mum would say to me "go in and have a look at what they have" – but I couldn't, I was completely unable to go into the pub on my own! I would always have to find an excuse, so that she would go in to look.

As I have no friends to go around with, if I don't go to places on my own, then I don't go at all. This means that I often have to fight myself, and go on my own. I will buy a ticket to events, knowing that when the occasion arrives, I will feel sick, but I endeavour to make myself go.

I do most of my 'fighting', when not fighting myself, by writing letters, or emails. My first big fight was to get a student grant to go to the Polytechnic of Wales, after the first college course I tried, turned into one of the disasters of my lifetime. This meant I needed a discretionary grant, which was very rarely given. A solicitor I then knew through the local church which I attended, helped me write a letter to apply for the grant. I then had to wait to see if my application was successful. Naturally, time when on, and I didn't hear anything. As July went into August, and the course started in September, I started to panic. I started ringing the council grant department every couple of days, to see if they had heard anything. On one occasion, I heard the girl who answered the phone saying "It's that Lynne (maiden name) on the phone again !!" in a resigned tone. I got my grant ! I have always thought it was due to persistence and wearing them down!

I have won many fights since, mostly with the local council, fighting for my sons. This started when Rhodri needed to go to a residential school. I had heard of children going to residential schools, but they were always older. Someone had told me they couldn't go until they were 11 years old. Rhodri was then 6 years old, and I didn't know how I was going to cope that long. I mentioned my plans to his social worker, who said that primary aged children could also go to residential schools.

I then researched suitable residential schools, and visited some with my Mum. We visited a lovely school in Blandford Forum "The Forum School". On sight, I knew it was the school for Rhodri, as it had a high fence round the grounds, and the playground had one approximately the height of a fence round a tennis court. The staff also said they would be able to toilet train him, as they had never had anyone who they couldn't train before – although most of their students were wearing nappies when they started. Other schools I visited said they wouldn't be able to do this. (Rhodri was toilet trained within one term of starting at the school!)

So, we started the fight! Many, many letters! At the start, I was unable to begin a letter, although I was fine at what to write once started. This was similar to my problems with talking. My Mum helped me with the letters because, working for the council (although a different department), she had an idea of how they should be written. When we began this fight, not many people had email, so I would email those councillors who did, as this would make my communications stand out. Nowadays, I write letters, as everyone else emails!

It took about two years, with letters to the education department, the chief executive of the council, councillors on the social services and education committees, a press release leading to articles in three local newspapers and an appearance on the local ITV news, and a very helpful correspondence with the Department of Education in London. In the end Rhodri received his funding for a place at the Forum School.

Unfortunately, as Rhodri got older, we needed more than the 38 week care, provided by the Forum School and he needed to change schools. The next school which did 50 week care, was a complete disaster for him. They had no understanding of his diet and needs, despite having agreed them before he started, which meant he was soon on the move again. There was less of a fight this time, as the council also wanted him to move, due to the residential school not keeping to their contract, and Rhodri was able to receive a place at "St Christopher's School" in Bristol, which provided 52 week care. He was very happy there, only leaving aged 18 to go to a residential care home.

This was naturally another fight, although less of one!
I researched and found a suitable home, which had a space available that would suit Rhodri. The council seemed to think that supported living would be ideal for him. However, Rhodri was soon moving to a lovely care home in Weston.

In between fighting for Rhodri's residential placements, I have also had fights for Bryn's school placements and for a residential college for him. Also, I fought the NHS for my friend, Steve, when he was in hospital long-term, and for a disabled facilities grant for him. I try not to have two fights at the same time, and have usually managed to alternate. However, I spent many years, when I was always fighting for something. Writing letters became normal, and now I'm writing this book!

My guide to fighting is this:

1. <u>Decide what you want !</u>

   This seems obvious, but surprisingly some people don't seem to know what they actually want to achieve. It is necessary to also find out if it is possible. Fighting for the impossible is a waste of time, and people will not take you seriously on future occasions. If you win once, then future fights are easier.

2. <u>Write Letters !</u>

   Don't phone! You can't prove your phone call. The person you phone may not write down what you actually say. A note on the file saying 'Mrs X phoned' says nothing. Send letters recorded delivery, so you can prove they got there, or hand deliver to the council offices (or whoever you are fighting) and ask for a receipt. They sometimes give you a photocopy, with a receipt stamp on it, what better way of proving that you wrote and what you said! If you need to phone, then follow up with a letter to the person to whom you spoke, saying "with reference to our telephone conversation on _____ I am writing to confirm _____ , stating whatever was said in the telephone call.

3. <u>Go Higher !</u>

   If you do not get the reply you want from your first correspondence, write to the manager of the department, and after that to the chief executive of the council/organisation. Research what their code of practice says about length of time they have to reply to you, and see that you get a reply in the time stated, otherwise send a copy of your letter to the next in line.

4. <u>Be Polite but Persistent !</u>

   This is the main thing to remember. Keep calm, which is easier by letter than by a phone call, and don't take 'no' for an answer. What usually happens is first you ask, they say 'no', if you then say 'ok' and leave it, then you only have yourself to blame. Unfortunately there is not enough money for everyone to have everything they want. If you think you have the right to what you need, then you will have to fight, and be the one who gets it. So, when they say 'no', appeal by writing!

5. <u>Know the Law and Quote it !</u>

   This is a lot easier now, due to the law and codes of practice etc, usually being on the internet. This part used to involve lots of reading in the central library! In your letter, quote the relevant regulation and what they need to do to keep to it.

M is for Meltdown

I don't really like the term 'meltdown', as unlike an ice cream, no-one is melting. Therefore I prefer to use the term 'panic attack' as I feel that this is more appropriate.

Panic is when I have been told off for doing something wrong.
Panic is when I have been confronted in a new situation, and have been unable to find words to express myself.
Panic is when I sit and cry, when I retreat into myself.
Panic is when I am unable to go out, and want to curl up in bed all day.
Panic is when I sit at the computer and play FreeCell (patience card game) for hours.
Panic is the result of fear and confusion.

When Bryn has a 'panic attack' he howls, makes dreadful looking faces, bangs his head with his hands, waves them around and leaps up and down. This is distressing to see, and frightening for people who have not seen this type of behaviour before and know little about autism. As he is over 6 ft tall, he towers over most people. At this time, it is pointless trying to ask questions. He already has too much going round in his mind and is overloaded with emotions. Adding your questions to the 'mess' in his mind will only add more confusion to the situation. I have found it better to check for injuries, and any obvious triggers. In his case, 'insects' e.g. flies etc, flying round him, would be a trigger and removing the fly would help him calm.

If there is no obvious solution, and he is not injured in any way that can be seen, I have always found it best to 'leave him to it', providing of course that he is in a safe environment such as his room, or a quiet area if away from home. Left in peace without being stared at, and being asked questions, is the best way for him to calm down. The same is true for me – having questions asked when I am in a panic, will lead to me giving wrong or misleading answers, simply because my mind is going down a different track.

My method generally with people having an autistic 'panic attack' is to ask myself the following questions.

<u>Are they seriously hurting themselves</u>?
Bryn presumably hurts himself when he bangs his head with his hand, but it's not the same type of injury as banging against a wall, and I have never known him to have a bruise afterwards.
<u>Are they hurting other people?</u>
<u>Are they breaking objects belonging to other people?</u>
<u>Are they breaking expensive objects belonging to themselves (that can't easily be replaced)?</u>
This would not count a magazine, etc. They could purchase another, and may possibly later learn from the experience.

If the answer to the four above questions is "No" and they <u>are</u> in a safe place, then my action will always be to 'leave them to it' and wait for them to calm before asking questions and trying to sort the problem.

Phobias may also lead to a panic attack. In the same way that one of my 'rules' is: "Don't start a routine, unless you want to be stuck in it", another rule is "Stop a phobia before it starts, or in the early stages". When a traumatic experience has happened, I try to erase memories from my mind, and sometimes I get a sense of panic when something reminds me of the event.

For example: A 'friend' decided she no longer wished to be friends with me, after being a large part of my life for over ten years. The cutting of the connection caused me much pain and distress. I found that even seeing a road sign pointing to the town in which she lived, sent panic rising through my body. I was unable to simply drive another way, as I had done in a similar situation in the past, as it was on the way to my son's care home and another route would take too long.

So I needed to find a way to desensitize myself to the signs, so that seeing them would not remind me of my 'friend' and the world I had lost. I had been looking for a group to join, or a craft class to attend to hopefully make a new friend. My Mum had mentioned that she had been to a talk by the owner of a craft shop in the town in question, and that they held craft courses. I felt at the time she told me, that it just shows that she doesn't know me at all, as she thought I could just go to the place as if nothing had happened. Her only remark was that it was a pity it wasn't nearer home.

However, I knew that I had to get over my increasing phobia about the town in general, so I decided that perhaps attending some of their courses would be a good idea. I looked on the internet and two sounded interesting. I know I daren't book online, I had to see if I could actually talk myself into driving into the town, let alone getting out of the car.

I was helped by the fact that the shop was at the opposite end of the town to where my 'friend' lived, and from other friends of hers that I knew. So, one day, on the way back from seeing my son, I drove to the shop and with great trepidation, as I don't usually feel able to go to new places on my own, I went in. I was fortunate that the shop had a large window frontage, so I could see most of the shop from the outside, this always makes me more able to enter new places.

I booked a place on two courses, and bought some craft materials, then went back to the car and drove home, feeling that I had made a start. For the first course, I simply drove to the shop, and went home afterwards. For the second, which was in the afternoon, I decided I would branch out further and go for a walk in the morning.

I had decided that I would visit a local tourist attraction. I had been there before with Rhodri and Steve years ago. I thought I would be safe from meeting anyone who knew me, as natives of an area normally don't frequent these types of places. It wasn't a very good day, damp and misty, but I sat watching the birds for a while. An older lady spoke to me saying "Good Morning" and commenting on the weather. She asked if I was local, and I explained that I was visiting for a craft course. She then said she lived opposite the attraction – so much for my idea that local people would be unlikely to visit!

I walked back to the shop without a problem and had a wonderful afternoon making beads from oven-bake clay at my course in the afternoon. I decided I had found a new craft to do! There will be other courses in a few months and I feel that I will be able to attend with ease. I can now see a road sign without a feeling of panic, and can remember the lovely time I had at the shop and watching the birds.

I'm sometimes asked how I can have Asperger's Syndrome when I don't throw myself on the ground and thrash about, or hit someone, when I have a meltdown/ panic attack. All I can say is that corporal punishment had not entirely died out when I was at school, and other punishments were more severe than being given a few days off school, which happens at the moment. My Mum was also expert at a hard slap across the top of the legs so, like others of my generation, I learnt other ways to cope!

REMEMBER

MY RULE NUMBER ONE

IF YOU DON'T WANT TO GET STUCK
IN A ROUTINE OR PATTERN,
DON'T MAKE IT ONE!

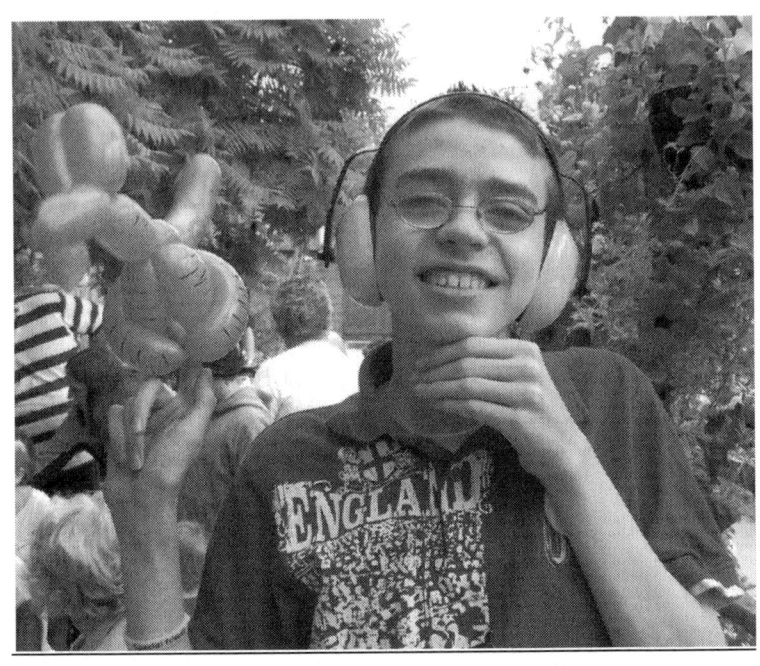

Brynmor is wearing his ear protectors. See page 97

N IS FOR 'NORMAL'

What is 'Normal'? Is anyone 'Normal'? Doesn't everyone have their own idiosyncrasies ?

In the autistic world, many people think 'Normal' is 'Not Autistic'. When I first began using the internet (in approximately 1994) I joined an Autism forum where most of the members were in the USA. At this time, I learnt to use the term Neuro-Typical (NT) for non-autistics, and this still seems to be fairly widely used today.

One of my favourite phrases at the moment seems to be "I don't do normal". I've had several builders doing alterations to my home, and keep hearing the words "It's normal to ......" usually describing what I don't want done. I end up saying look " I don't do normal, there are two autistics in this house, 'normal' we are not!"

I wish that other people would understand, that if someone has an Autistic Spectrum Disorder, it doesn't make them not a person like everyone else.

People with autism are people first – having the same feelings, body and basic needs (warmth, food etc..) as everyone else. On an internet forum recently, there was a discussion started by someone who had a partner with Asperger's Syndrome, who said she couldn't cope with his behaviour.

The resulting discussion from various members of the forum, seemed to be saying that people with Asperger's were a different species and not a person like everyone else. I don't understand this point of view, which I have seen & heard many times. Most people can be categorised in one way or other. E.g. Partially sighted people (anyone who wears glasses), Mobility impaired people, People with red hair ....

I can never understand why adults with a learning disability who live in a residential care home, are referred to as 'service users' of the home. Why? It's all very well to be a 'service user' of a day centre or support agency, but why when you live in a house are you called this term. Why not 'resident'? You can get residents of a block of flats, not 'service users of a block of flats'. Elderly people are 'residents' of nursing homes, why is it different for people with learning difficulties? To me, the term 'Service User' seems to emphasise the company/service, while 'resident' emphasises the person. When I worked in a nursing home, in 2005, we were instructed to say 'client' when talking about the people who lived there – but that is no better in my opinion.

Everyone is themselves, and has a right to individuality and to be treated as a human being.

O IS FOR ORGANISING

I like to think I'm a good organiser. I think attention to detail and logical thought is part of my Autism. I have been involved in organising fundraising events for many years. Even when at school, I organised a small summer fete in my garden at home one year, to raise money for my school, which had been destroyed by fire. I persuaded family and neighbour's children to look after stalls.

When I had left college, with an HND in Mathematics, Statistics & Computing, I was unable to find a job for a while. I was living back at home with my parents and hoped to make some friends locally. I thought about a computer club and wrote a piece for a 'The Foresters' local newsletter, asking if anyone would like to join one. This was an organisation with several different interest groups, and I thought a computer group would be a good idea. This was in 1982, so there weren't a lot of home computers around. I arranged a hall for a first meeting, to see if there was any response. Unfortunately for me, the only response was about seven children aged 10 – 12 years old, and only one adult – who seeing all the children made his escape quite quickly! So, instead of making friends of around my own age (22), I ended up starting a children's computer club, which turned into a general youth club with other activities such as table tennis as well as computers.

When Rhodri first went to residential school, I wanted find some activities in the school holidays for Bryn then aged 11. There was nothing suitable at the leisure centre etc. for an autistic 11 year old, who had the mind of a 5 year old, so I set about providing something myself. I distributed a questionnaire to parents through the local National Autistic Society group, and a local special school, asking if there were any other parents in my situation. Several parents contacted me, and having spoken to two leisure centres, I booked activities for the following summer holidays.

The club grew mostly from word of mouth, although I was able to get several press releases into the local papers, and I subsequently applied for registered charity and limited company status. Then, when my son was 14, I added a weekly youth club to the activities. Requests from parents of younger children caused a junior youth club to be formed. There was also an occasional club on Saturdays, meeting at a local activity centre providing adventurous activities e.g. climbing and archery.

When I left the charity as my sons became too old to attend a children's group, it had grown over six years from a membership of 15 children to 85 children, and from being completely self-funding by parents, to having an income of £20,000 a year from grants and other sources. I was pleased with the growth of the charity, and with what I had managed to achieve, mostly through my own efforts with minimal help.

When I felt I had finished writing this book, I thought about possible designs for the cover. Thinking that a photo of Brynmor, Rhodri and myself would be good, as the book is all about us, I went to look for one. Having discovered no suitable recent photograph, I decided to have one taken. All the photographs I already possessed had only one of my sons in them, and even earlier ones with two didn't have me in them, as I was taking the photos.

Therefore I needed to get all of us together, with someone else to take the photo. Most families would have no problem with taking a snapshot type photo of three of its members. However, for us it had to be a well-planned operation, started a week before.

Problems included Rhodri living in Weston, Bryn & I living in Bristol (about 30 miles apart). Bryn won't stay in the same room as Rhodri for more than about 10 seconds, won't even stay on the same floor as him at home and refuses to go anywhere near Rhodri's care home.

I decided that a photograph taken on Weston seafront would be best. I did get one of them on opposite ends of a seat there about 18 months previously, but that one had a shadow of me taking the photo so was no good for what we needed now.

So, I emailed the care home, saying I would take Rhodri out on the day in question, and if it was fine, we would be taking his photo so asked that he was wearing tidy clothes. We always go out with a support worker from the home in case of any problem with his behaviour.

I arranged to take Bryn & <u>his</u> support worker to Weston, and while I went to collect Rhodri they walked down to the shops. I found Rhodri was wearing a limp black t-shirt, however I had taken a new t-shirt with me for him to wear, as I knew that my hope of him wearing something tidy and suitable for a photograph would not happen. Then I phoned Bryn's support worker on the way down to the sea, to tell them to go to the pier and wait for us. What did we do before mobile phones?

We sat on the sea wall by the pier, and surprisingly Brynmor & Rhodri seemed to enjoy having their photo taken, with me sat between them. I gave my ipod touch to one support worker, and camera to the other, and between them they took thirty photos, in the hope that in one of them we would all be looking nice. With two people taking photographs we became a subject of interest to people passing by, and my sons seemed to enjoy the attention, unlike me! You can see the result on the cover! I have decided that the ipod touch is brilliant for taking photos of autistic people, as it takes lots of pictures one after another, rather than the camera which seems to take ages to save one photo before being ready to take another.

You may think that this is a lot of organisation just to take a snapshot type photograph!

P IS FOR PROSOPAGNOSIA

Prosopagnosia is an impairment that results in an inability to remember faces. A lot of people with Autism and Asperger's Syndrome, have difficulty with this. I just can't remember who people are. I know I should know someone, if they address me by my name – but I haven't a clue who they are, I used to say hello and "can't stop" and leave quickly, but now I just ask them to remind me who they are, and I have to put up with the odd looks.

I sometimes have extremely embarrassing moments when someone I know well (often even people I see 2 or 3 times a week) has his or her hair cut – and I don't recognise him or her – I see a stranger. It's only when they talk (I'm best at voices) that I recognise them. So if I see a stranger, in a place where I normally know everyone, I don't ask anyone who it is, but wait to see if I actually know him or her anyway, particularly if no-one else shows surprise that they are there.

Research has shown that people with Asperger's Syndrome, process faces in a different part of their brain to other people. We remember faces in the same way as inanimate objects, while other people have a different section of their brain for remembering faces.

I remember people by their hairstyle, clothes, the way they move, their voice etc. but not by their faces. I have even not recognised my family on occasions.

IT WORKED FOR US!

In 1994, using public toilets became difficult with a 5 and 3 year old, neither of whom could be left outside the cubicle. Changing a 3 yr olds nappy on the floor in the ladies wasn't great either. I was able to purchase a key for the disabled toilets from RADAR (www.radar-shop.org.uk).

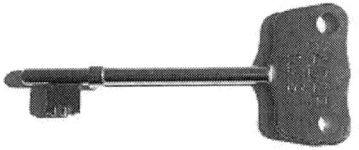

Rhodri still uses his RADAR key, as it is safer for him, and the general public, if he can use the disabled toilet. Especially when he needs 'time out', when he is anxious. He can then be on his own at this time, to enable himself to calm.

PROBLEM SOLVED !

Q IS FOR QUESTIONS

This is a plea on behalf of all autistic people particularly children, don't make something a question if it isn't one!

For example:

Don't say "shall we go shopping now?"
What do you say when the child answers "no"?
If you mean "we are going shopping" - say so!

Although, with Brynmor, I would need to agree a time to go shopping, e.g. "what time shall we go shopping?" We can negotiate a time, but the shopping is definitely happening!

or:

"Would you like to sit down?" usually just means "sit down"

Say what you mean. People have told me that they are trying to be polite by making it a question. You are being more polite to autistic people, if you say what you mean, so they are not confused.

I have a problem with other types of questions, an example:

"Would you like a cup of coffee?"

It will seem a simple question to most people but my problem is I don't like coffee, but I would like a cup of tea. So I think –

Do I say "No thank you"? (I don't want a cup of coffee)
Do I say " No thank you, I don't like coffee"?
Would this person mind if I say "Can I have tea?" or "Do you have any tea?"
These worries go round and round in my mind.

In the end usually I will say "No thank you", unless I know the person well, in which case I will ask if I can have tea.

I also hate the question "why". It's not a question I use very often. If I ask someone if they are going to a certain event, and they say "no", then I accept that. It doesn't usually occur to me to ask "why". If I thought about it at all, I would think that it was none of my business, and if the person wanted me to know, they would have told me.

My Mum has always reprimands me, if she asks for example: "is X going to the meeting?" If I said "no", she would say "why not?" And I would say "I don't know, she didn't say". Mum always says "didn't you ask?"

It was only after I began to meet more people that I discovered the problem of the "why" question. Part of the problem, is that I don't tell lies. Actually I can tell lies, but I generally have to practise what I'm going to say in advance, I'm not very good at 'spur of the moment' lies. So if I'm suddenly asked for example: "why are you not doing ...." And I don't want to answer, then I have a problem. The person asking me keeps asking why – and I don't know what to say. It's back to the 'empty rooms' in the chapter 'C for Conversation'.

So either:
I'm pressurised into telling the truth – which ends up with me, and possibly other people, being upset.
Or
My upsetting the questioner, as I tell them to mind their own business.

I now have some set answers along the lines of "I'm sorry, I can't tell you that" in the case of my not breaking a confidence, or more usually " I don't know" , even when I <u>do</u> know. The set answer for when I'm not going somewhere is, "I can't get a sitter/childcare" – but I think a lot of people use that excuse!

As a child I found it was necessary to tell a lie to keep to 'rules' (see page 15) with regard to saying "thank you, that's nice", for gifts, even if I didn't like them. Also, when agreeing, when it wasn't what I actually thought, but because that is the easier option and won't get me into trouble. I decided as a child that a 'yes' or 'no' on its own isn't a lie, just keeping people happy.

Bryn does this too, a 'yes' or 'no' from him may be the right answer for what he thinks, but may not, it may just be an automatic answer just to keep the questioner quiet. But an actual sentence will always be the truth.

When I am extremely stressed, perhaps because of changes in my life that I can't control, I go into "autistic mode". I can often feel this coming on, but have difficulty stopping it happening. If I go into a "tunnel of hell" (see H is for Hell) then it's too late – I am in "autistic mode", and will stay there for months, gradually climbing out.

One of my problems during this time, is that I am unable to ask strangers questions. I went shopping with my paraplegic friend, Steve, during an "autistic mode" recently, to buy him a lap tray he needed. Visiting a large department store near his home, we were unable to find the trays. Steve said "Ask that assistant over there", but I made him go to ask.

This is something I had never been able to do before I learnt conversation and some sociability. I'm normally able to do this now but the problems come back during an "autistic mode" and I am back where I was before. I wander round and round supermarkets, particularly when they have decided to move all the goods around, and recently being unable to find the bacon, I went without rather than approach an assistant, as thought of this solution made me feel ill.

I have noticed my need to keep up skills, in order not to lose them. When I was away at college, I learnt confidence to go to new places on my own, but after leaving college and moving back with my parents, I was unable to keep up with this skill and lost the ability.

While at work, I learnt to use the phone with confidence, even helping out on the switchboard in the lunchtimes at one job. However, when I left work having given birth to Bryn, I had no real practice using phones (other than talking to my Mum), so I lost that skill. I'm slightly better if it is a professional phone call – i.e. I am talking on behalf of someone else or an organisation, but I dislike making personal phone calls and have to save them up for a day that I am feeling more confident. I always try to find an email address for any communications I have to make, and organisations who insist on phone calls always annoy me.

My phone calls tend to only be practical – I say the minimum possible. For example, if I'm phoning to arrange to meet someone. After the person answered the phone, I will say "it's Lynne", and they answer "oh, hello" or similar. I will say "can I come to see you on Tuesday", they would say yes/no, possibly mention another day and we would arrange a time. Then I would say thank you and end the call. I wouldn't have been able to find anything else to talk about.

Any social skills I had managed to gain during college and work, were lost when I was at home after having my children. My husband worked permanent nights, for six nights a week and stayed up for the seventh, as he didn't want his body clock to have to change. So, I didn't see him much. If he wasn't in bed asleep, he was out. I had no-one else to talk to, and used to go to the local Tesco most days, if only to have a conversation with the girl on the till. I couldn't initiate conversation, but often they were friendly and asked something about my children, or commented on the weather etc.

Bryn would mainly only go to sleep by the movement of the pushchair or the car, so we went for lots of walks or drives. We would often catch a bus, or train. Now, as an adult, Bryn has to show his support workers how to catch a train – having been doing so regularly since he was about 6 weeks old!

I remember being in high spirits (for me) for days, after a guard on the train had been kind to me and held up the train, while he helped me carry my tandem pushchair up the steps to leave the station. It was a small unmanned station on a local line, with only the two platforms, and level access on only one side. In those days, people with pushchairs, particularly large double/tandem ones, could travel in the guard's van and had no need to remove the children from the pushchair during the journey. I had been trying to get Bryn (who was a toddler) to get out in order that he could walk up the steep steps, so I could bump up Rhodri (who was a baby) in the pushchair. Bryn was too heavy for me to get both of them up the steps in the chair. He was tired and didn't want to walk so was hanging on, thereby refusing to get out by action, if not by speech. The guard came and said "I'll give you a hand" and moved to lift the front of the pushchair, I said "What about the train?" and he said "It can wait"!

R IS FOR ROUTINES AND RULES

People on the autistic spectrum always like routines. Doing things the same way, at the same time gives a calming and safe feeling. It's about 'needing to know' what is happening next. We don't like sudden changes, as our brains are not wired up for them.

I always say "Never start a routine, if you don't want to get stuck in it!". Knowing what is going to happen is the key to autistic people's lives. However, in some situations a routine may cause a problem. Later in this chapter, I describe how a routine inadvertently started that almost made Bryn only attend school on four days each week! Routines that can't accept actions such as shops closing down, road works etc. will also cause problems.

This is an example I give to people to explain about routines:

"Imagine you are having an autistic child for tea for a number of weeks. Perhaps it's a friend's child, who needs a break. The child comes after school, and you give him sausage and chips for tea. All well you think. The next week, sausages are on offer in the supermarket again, and he liked them didn't he? So you serve sausage and chips for tea again. The following week, beefburgers are on offer – you can't understand why this child is screaming "sausages!" and refusing to eat – but the routine of sausage and chips for tea at your house has been started! If there was sausage & chips the first week, beef burgers and chips the next, and something else with chips the third, then you will be stuck with the chips, but able to have a variety of other foods with them!"

When I gave birth to Bryn, people kept telling me that I needed to get him into a routine. I didn't understand what I was supposed to do, in order to start this routine. Especially since Bryn only slept for about 8 hours in 24 in two hours slots, but not at the same time each day. I kept asking these people what they meant, what extra was I supposed to do to be a "routine"? I have realised since, that I was already doing my own 'routine' without knowing it, and so adding to it to conform with this request was impossible. I didn't know that everyone wasn't born with this need to do things the same way etc, until I was diagnosed with Asperger's Syndrome and went to talks about Autism and found out that I was the one who was 'different'.

Brynmor especially has had a lot of routine behaviours over the years. All children mature, autistic children are not immune from this, and so the routine behaviours that occurred when they were 6 years old, are not likely to be the same as when they are 16 years. This is the case for Bryn anyway. It annoyed me when he was at primary school, when the teacher complained at a review meeting, about one of his behaviours at the time, age 6. I have forgotten what exactly it was, only that it was normal behaviour for 3 year olds, which was the age he was mostly functioning at the time. She said "you don't want him to be doing it when he is 16", so he was to be stopped from doing it now. I pointed out he was 6! He had ten years to go until he was 16! This is one example of many occasions when Bryn wasn't expected to behave as a child, but as an adult while at primary school! I can never understand the reasoning of this, surely it is healthier to go through all the stages of growing up, even if at a different age to 'most people'. I believe in letting children be children, and I didn't stop Bryn from doing the behaviour – which he soon grew out of anyway!

I have found it necessary to think carefully before trying to change behaviour that I may think unsuitable – Does it really do any harm to anyone? When behaviours are stopped, others take their place and often I have found I wished the first one back – as the new one is worse!

Some annoying behaviours are learnt from others. Bryn aged about 7, started cutting fabric that hung e.g. curtains, tablecloths – which was very annoying. If he managed to get his hands on a pair of scissors, there would be a chunk taken out of something. He managed to do some damage with a table knife too. At a school review meeting, the teacher asked if he had any behaviours at home which concerned me, and I mentioned this new fascination with cutting curtains etc.. The classroom assistant exclaimed "Oh Dear!", we all turned to look at her and she reminded the teacher that when they decided the curtains in the classroom were too long, she cut them off at the windowsills, while they were hanging, and later took them home to sew. This had happened twice, for different windows, while the children were in the room! Bryn fortunately grew out of that behaviour too, but only after all my tablecloths were in shreds!

With practice, autistic people can learn to cope with some changes in routine. When Brynmor was first diagnosed, my husband went to the library and borrowed most of the books on autism. I discovered through reading these, that there were lots of autistic children who would only go in shops in the same order, only travel to places by the same route etc. I realised that this would be a problem – suppose a shop closed down? Or road works meant a diversion? I was determined that Brynmor (and later, Rhodri) would not be like that, so I didn't follow the same route every time. Sometimes we have just 2 or 3 routes, and I will say "we will go this way today". If you don't get into a 'pattern', then you won't have to stay in that 'pattern'.

I was shown this was correct when, one January when taking Rhodri back to his residential school (aged 8). He had been asking to go back for days, by putting his uniform on – in the end, I had to hide it until the day school started back! Recent heavy snow storms, meant that the area we usually drove through was blocked. Unusually for me, we had always gone the same way to his school 60 miles away from home – It was the only way I knew and I didn't get lost. However, on this occasion, we had to get the map out, and find a new way. We wondered why Rhodri was creating havoc in the back of the car – kicking, pulling my hair (I was driving!), and biting my mum who was trying to read the map. We eventually got on our usual route and the havoc in the back stopped abruptly and Rhodri was all smiles and making his happy noises. Mum & I were wrecks! I now <u>always</u> have more than one regular way to go to places!

I do feel stressed, if one of my 'patterns' changes, but it would only usually make me a bit 'off', not quite right. It feels a bit like 'butterflies' in my stomach, a slightly nauseous feeling. Other people do not normally notice. Unless there are several changes at the same time, or if I am particularly stressed, when I may 'lose it' and shout at someone. If autistic children have sudden changes, it could cause a severe tantrum and possibly them attacking themselves or someone else. However teenagers and adults who have never had to cope with changes at an early age, are also severely affected later in life.

I always find myself parking in about the same place in a car park. If asked why, I would say it's so I can find my car. That's not the real problem, as it is an unusual colour, but I feel embarrassed saying that it makes me feel peculiar if I park in the 'wrong' place. I also tend to sit in the same chair at meetings. I have to get there early, due to not being able to walk into a crowded room, so I can usually get the same seat or the at least the same area of the hall. More than about half a dozen people is 'crowded' in this instance, less if it's a small room. If something happened and I had to sit on the 'wrong' side, I would feel 'out of sorts' for the whole meeting.

There are times when routines are useful. When Bryn started nursery school, I was always worried about him escaping, and coming home. This was before any of us were diagnosed autistic. My natural thought was to always walk the same way to/from nursery school, using the zebra crossing, which was on a very clear part of the road, where it is easy to see anyone crossing. This meant we only crossed one other road, which was a quiet cul-de-sac. Other people didn't seem to understand my insistence that having always gone that way, Bryn would go that way if he 'escaped'. It always seemed logical to me!

Once, I was in our local shopping centre with Bryn. I sent him to post some letters while I was at the cash point – I try to give him some jobs to do independently. He didn't return from the nearby post-box, so I walked round the corner to it – no Bryn! I hung around for a while, before dialling 999 (which was always my immediate reaction, when my children were younger and missing) and he soon reappeared coming from the wrong direction. I said "where have you been?" and he said "Post Office". He had obviously misunderstood my instruction. As his trip had meant crossing two main roads, I was glad we <u>always</u> use the crossings on the traffic lights!

I am concerned when I read these days, that when parents are told their child has an autistic spectrum disorder and find they don't like change – they don't give them any! How is that helping anyone long term? Children learn things easier than adults, so the time to learn that 'change happens and you will have to learn to cope with it' is when you are young. It is helpful if you can still pick the child up and move them bodily if necessary. By forcing some change on autistic children, they will come to be used to the situation occurring. Having a teenager/adult who can't accept any changes and makes up all the rules is no help to either themselves or anyone else.

One Monday morning when Bryn was 12, he told me "no school" when I went to wake him. He was normally correct when he indicated he was ill by saying these words, so I cancelled the taxi that took him to school. He woke up later, and seemed fine – which surprised me. The next Monday he said "no school" again. At the time, I had forgotten about the week before, due to the stress of other things happening, so again he stayed home, and again he seemed fine. The following week was half term, during the week he kept saying "no school on Monday". I kept saying Yes, there was school on Mondays, not on Saturdays or Sundays.

Then I had a brainwave! At the beginning of the month there had been the May Bank Holiday when the school was only shut for one day. I realised that the teachers had impressed on the children that there was "no school on Monday"! I really wish these people would think before they speak! If they had said "no school on Monday 7th May", I wouldn't now have this problem.

Well, it was either having a child who only went to school four days a week, or forcing the issue. The routine of no school on Mondays was now in evidence, so it was necessary to break it. On the Monday morning, I forcibly got Bryn out of bed, dressed him and as he refused to get in the taxi, put him in the back of my car and drove him the ten miles to school! There I dragged him in, gave a quick explanation to a teacher, put him in a classroom, closed the door and got out quick!! It was their problem now, and was of their making anyway! The following Monday, he went to school on the taxi as usual!

Rhodri & I normally have an usual route for our walks around Weston, which involves going to the indoor shopping centre, visiting the toilet, before going to Tesco, then returning to his care home. One morning, I was surprised when Rhodri suddenly led me down a side street, where we hadn't been together before. He always decides where we are going, but the route rarely deviates very much, and then only to include the pier. He then proceeded to walk through the back streets, to the other end of the high street, and we approached the indoor centre from the opposite way to usual. I must admit to getting my 'odd' feeling, due to the change. Half way round the indoor shopping centre, I found myself suggesting to Rhodri, that perhaps we could go to Tesco as usual, as I didn't really like the change. He turned us round (he holds my arm) and we walked back the other way towards Tesco, incidentally bumping into his support workers who were following us. They asked what was happening and I said that I hadn't liked the change, so Rhodri was taking me back to our usual route! Having taught my sons to accept change – I can't do it myself!

In common with most autistic people, I generally keep to rules. I can break rules but I always feel very guilty. If I do something that I know is against the rules, I always get very worried about it and often have a sick feeling in my stomach. I don't like being reminded of when I have done wrong.

I read an article on the National Autistic Society website about an autistic spectrum condition called PDA (Pathological Demand Avoidance), which says that people with the condition want other people to follow rules but don't keep to the same rules themselves. I have known several children diagnosed with Asperger's syndrome who do this and never understood why they don't keep to the rules that they expect other people to do. I had thought that this was a side effect of the 'I have special needs syndrome', as several children have told me that "the rule" was that they didn't have to keep to "the rules that everyone else did" as they "have special needs"!

However, it seems that PDA is a separate condition and not Asperger's Syndrome, although part of the autistic spectrum. More information can be found on the National Autistic Society Website at: www.autism.org.uk

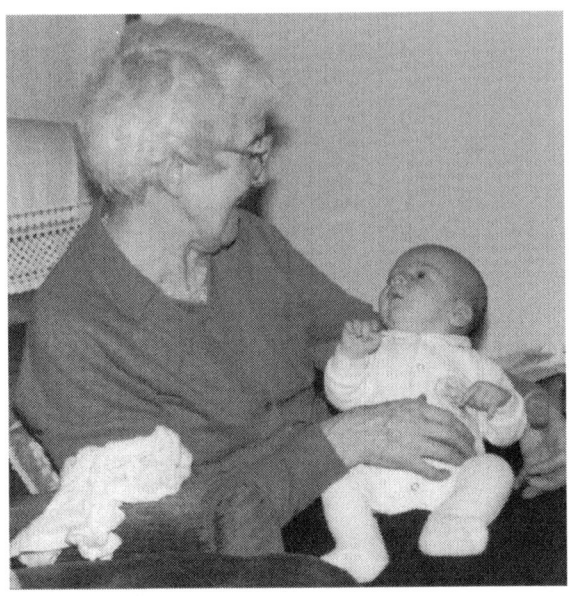

Rhodri (aged 8 weeks) is showing his gazing at faces behaviour, which always made me feel so uncomfortable. (see page 38). Here he is pictured with his great-grandma.

S IS FOR SENSITIVITIES

Both my sons are highly sensitive to sound. Bryn can hear talking in the kitchen, when he is in his bedroom with the door shut. I only have to say "Tea's ready" in a normal voice, and he comes (providing he's not playing his music extremely loudly). He spends most of his time wearing noise reduction earplugs, and in very noisy situations, ear defenders as well. I have recently discovered that it is possible to buy child sized ear defenders, I wish I knew that when my sons were small, although possibly they didn't make them then!

When Bryn was seven years old, we fundraised to take him for Auditory Integration Training in London, a two week course. This involved him listening to specially recorded music through headphones for half an hour twice a day. It worked by desensitising the ear to certain frequencies that were causing problems.

Before we went, I would have to walk miles to circumvent road works etc, when out. After the course, I found I could walk past the road works without having a screaming child. It was actually like he 'woke up' at two years old. We had the 'terrible two's' again, he answered "no" to every question. How I longed for a "yes"! Eventually it happened, which was wonderful. At that period in time, my Mum (who hadn't heard a yes before) took Bryn into a baker's shop and asked if him if he would like a bun. He said "yes" and she was so pleased, telling him how good he was. Another customer made a remark about 'children these days not saying please' and my Mum, pointed out that he was autistic and he normally said 'no' to everything. Unfortunately the effect of the A.I.T. treatment has worn off over the years, and he has become very sensitive to sound again.

Both my sons hate people talking about them, without them being included. As both also have this extremely sensitive hearing, they can hear you talking about them from quite a distance. Actually I hadn't really understood how much they can hear, until Steve (a self-diagnosed Aspie) lived with us for a while. His hearing is also extremely acute, and he was continually complaining about dogs barking etc, that I couldn't hear. Once I went in search of this dog, and found the noise came from a house halfway down the street. As all our double glazed windows were shut at the time, and anyway, I couldn't hear it from out in the garden, this was a surprise. I came to realise that my sons have this acute hearing too.

My sons and I are all unhappy in crowds. The noise is one problem, and the closeness of other people. It's also easy to lose each other in a crowd. I have lost Bryn several times in busy shopping areas, necessitating in an appeal to security or phoning 999 – depending on whether it was an enclosed shopping mall, or on a high street. He was once lost for hours one Christmas Time. Bryn didn't seem concerned when he was eventually tracked down by police and collected by me from the security office of a music store, but I was a wreck! When

I lost him in Bath town centre (he had 'disappeared' while I was choosing something to buy), I was surprised by the number of local people, even local tourist guides, who did not know the location of the police station! He turned up in a music store again on that occasion. I had checked the store on the way to the police station, but he must have been hidden somewhere, as I hadn't seen him.

These days, I don't tend to lose him. He has stopped wandering off, although he does go off to the toilet without saying where he is going. He does now come back, if I wait around where I last saw him. My main worry is if he is approached by someone. Bryn has reasonable commonsense. However, he is unlikely to understand if anyone speaks to him, to give instructions e.g. not to go into a certain part of a store that is closed, and he could easily be taken by anyone. If they said "come with me" he would go. When he was a child, I often found him trying to leave a shop with groups of adults and children. The adults having said something like "right we are going now, come this way" and he would be trying to go too! Thinking they were speaking to him!

Once I lost both of them at the same time. It was when Bryn suddenly learnt how to open the front door. I was cooking tea and felt a breeze. I dashed to the front door and Bryn was on the pavement and Rhodri not anywhere to be found. I frantically dialled 999. The police wanted to know what he was wearing, this was a t-shirt and a nappy – and nothing else! They insisted on knowing the colour of the t-shirt, they apparently couldn't report him lost without this information, but in my panic I couldn't remember. Finally, I decided to just pick a colour and said "red", then they said they would put out a call for the police to look for him.

I had a phone call, fifteen minutes or so later. A member of the public had phoned them to tell them about a child wearing only a t-shirt (he had removed the nappy) who was balancing on a ledge over the dual carriage way. This doesn't bear thinking about! When he was returned to me in the police car, his t-shirt turned out to be blue! It seems that the police were able to recognise him despite the wrong colour t-shirt! Rhodri didn't seem at all concerned about having been lost, he was smiling away in the police car. I had been cooking cheese sauce at the time when they escaped. It was many years before I could bring myself to cook cheese sauce again!

Bryn has a sensitivity to light, especially sunlight. He often closes the curtains of his room. He used to get lots of headaches. The opticians suggested light sensitive lens for him, which would automatically shade in sunlight. This proved to be a success, and he is a lot happier outside now, and no longer gets headaches.

Rhodri is sensitive to heat. He gets extremely irritable if he is hot. He never seems to understand that he would be cooler if he took a layer of his clothes off. After being in the routine of wearing a jumper & jacket during the winter, he tries to wear them in the summer too. I have had a continual fight with residential schools who insist that Rhodri should wear what he chooses – which means he often came out wrapped up in a thick jumper on a hot day, while attacking me because he was hot! I just removed all the unnecessary clothes and he became very happy again! I was so sorry for him having to cope with the heat on the days that I was not there.

I've discovered that most people can tune into speech etc. and cut out the background noise. I can't, I hear all that too. In a meeting, I often can't hear what is being said, because of the noise of the air-conditioning, the tea urn, the traffic through the window etc. Regular noises annoy me. I can't sleep with a clock that ticks. If I'm away and there is one, I have to wrap it up in a large towel, or similar, and shut in a drawer, or I can still hear it.

When I discovered this is different for most other people, I got a flashback memory to a lesson when I was in the first year at secondary school (now year 7). I can't remember the subject, maybe English? We were asked to keep very quiet, and to listen for noises we didn't usually hear. At the end of five minutes or so, the teacher asked the class to put their hands up, if they heard something they didn't usually hear. All hands went up, except mine, so I eventually put my hand up, so as not to be different, although I didn't usually speak in class. Suggestions from the class were "the radiators knocking", "the birds", "the cars"... I thought they were cheating – those noises were always there. When asked what I had heard, I said the lorry reversing outside – after all, there wasn't permanently a lorry reversing outside!

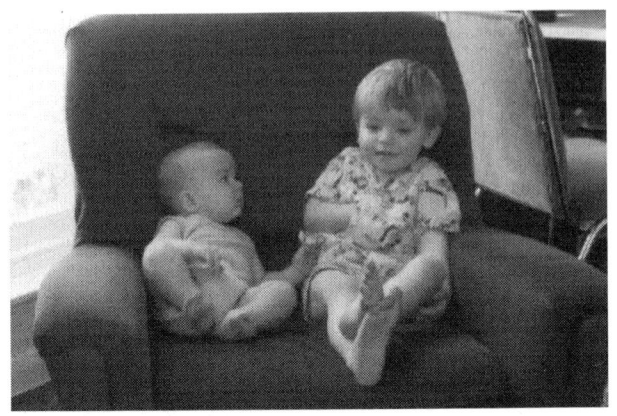

This is one of my favourite photographs of my boys. Rhodri was about 4 months and Bryn 2 years old.

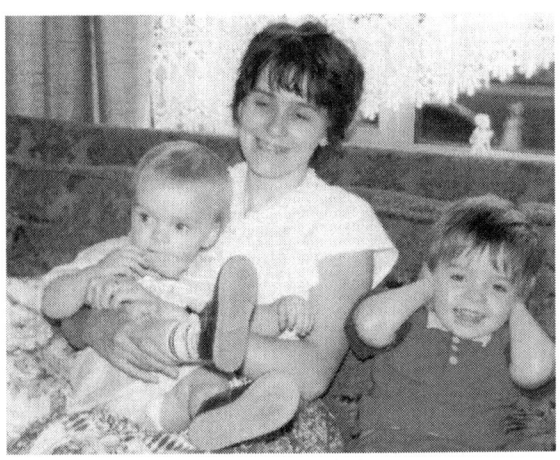

Taken a year later, Bryn shows that his sound sensitivity started at an early age, as did Rhodri's continual attempts to escape – most photos show me holding on firmly to him to keep him still.

T IS FOR TREATING PEOPLE LIKE PARCELS

There is a tendency amongst professionals to forget that people who are disabled, particularly with learning difficulties, are people with feelings. When my son came home from his residential school for holidays for a week or more, I needed respite care during the time he was home. When I was sent the date allocated for respite care, it was often the day after he came home, or once the same day! I had to refuse and was told that if I didn't accept that date, then I wouldn't get any more.

My son's social worker didn't seem to understand, why I was not prepared to accept this date. I asked her, as single mum, if she would want to send her daughter away the day after she came home, after 6 weeks away – wouldn't her daughter want to spend time with her mum, before going away again? I said that Rhodri was a person, having feelings, wanting his mum, not a parcel to be moved around without thought. She then understood my point, and we were given a date later in the holidays.

However this problem is one that I have seen in various forms many times over the years. Including, support workers walking with service users, who totally ignore the people they are supporting, looking bored to death, or texting or chatting on their mobiles. Rhodri hates people talking when he is not included. When visiting his school once with his social worker, we witnessed him going for a walk with two staff who were having a discussion over his head, and ignoring him. He was beginning to look stressed and his social worker went up to speak to them to point out that they should have been talking to Rhodri, not talking between themselves. I had to hide behind a tree, as if he saw me he would have wanted to go home! It's quite easy to talk to service users, pointing out flowers, cars, talking about where we are going, what we are going to do/see, what we will do when we get back. Autistic people in particular, need to know what is happening, especially in a new place, and often like to be reassured by being told the same things several times.

I have found that the best way to deal with children & adults who have a habit of suddenly sitting down when walking, e.g. on the pavement, is to sit down with them and stop conversation. Rhodri always used to do this, and I found that if I said "that's a good idea, I could do with a rest", sat down by him, and ignored him, then he would be up in no time and we would be off walking again. This experience came in useful, when I supported an adult who also did the same thing – I think she did it for attention, as other support workers tried to persuade her to get up, tried pulling her up, bribing etc. from which she would have gained a lot of amusement. As I stopped talking, which I had been doing whilst walking, and sat down by her, she decided not to bother doing it again with me – not so much fun!

Do you remember the Radio 4 programme "Does he take Sugar?" It was a programme for disabled people, referring to the habit of some people to refuse to address questions to them. The worst example I experienced of this type of behaviour, was when I accompanied my paraplegic friend, Steve, to a local health centre for a podiatry appointment. Due to his spinal injury and diabetes, he has to go there to have his toe nails cut. This was his first visit, and I had gone to help him get his wheelchair out of the car and hold it for him to get in, as the car park is on a steep slope. He was the driver of the car. Bryn had to come along, so the plan was that we would all go in (it being boring for us to stay in the car) and we would look at the magazines in the waiting room while Steve had his nails cut.

On arrival, we were met by the podiatrist who insisted that I accompany them both into the treatment room. I stated that I couldn't leave Bryn alone, so he had to come too. She appeared a bit 'put out' by this, but had no option but to agree. Then she proceeded to give me a form to complete. I didn't bother arguing about this, as I knew Steve would give it to me as my handwriting was more readable than his. Although, later I thought perhaps I should have confused her totally by giving the form to Bryn, who has the neatest writing of the three of us.

The podiatrist continued to ask me questions about my friend's foot care, how often he washes his feet etc. I naturally, had to ask him and he then replied. After a few questions, I got fed up and pointed out to her that it would save time if she asked Steve her questions directly, being that he was 50 years old with full mental faculties. I didn't bother pointing out that, although a self-diagnosed Aspie, he has more conversational abilities than me. I tend to try to hide behind him & his wheelchair, which is quite large as he was 6'4" tall when he could stand, and is over 20 stone, so being addressed by people who refuse to talk to him is annoying in the extreme.

I would really think that professionals working for the NHS would have sufficient disability awareness training to avoid this type of situation.

The opposite is a problem when someone, for instance staff at a bank, insist on talking to Bryn. Bryn answers "yes ok" to any questions that he doesn't understand, which are most questions put by strangers. I managed to solve this problem by having a joint account with him. He has a bank card, is the only one who knows his number, and can look at his account on the internet. However, having my name on the account means that I can ring if the card is lost and another needs to be ordered, otherwise the bank would need to receive the request from him and he could have agreed to anything with his "yes ok", even if I managed to get him to read the words "I have lost my card" etc from a piece of paper, down the phone.

U IS FOR UNDERSTANDING

Everyone always says that one of the standard 'symptoms' of Autism is 'lack of empathy'.

From a dictionary: Empathy - Identification with and understanding of another's situation, feelings, and motives.

I remember my Mum always telling me, when I couldn't understand someone's reaction to something, that I should think what I would feel in the same situation.

This type of empathy has become easier as I have got older, and had more experience of various situations myself. I find it easy to imagine what I would feel in a situation similar to one I have had in the past. However, I still find it very difficult if it's something I haven't experienced myself.

I am often amazed when it often seems that I (the autistic!) can understand another person's feelings, when other people seem unable to do so. An example of this is when I was volunteering in a local charity shop. A customer came to collect an item of furniture purchased previously. A manager asked me to help him take the item to her car. I could see (and hear) her baby crying in the car. I found the item and pointed it out to him. On his way to help me with it, he started tidying the display of other items. I reminded him we were taking the item of furniture out to a customer who was waiting in the car with her crying baby, and he carried on tidying the shelves, which could have been done at any time! I seemed to be the only one who could understand the frustration of the customer, and the need to be as quick as possible so she could get on her way home. My grandfather had a hardware shop, where my Mum & Dad worked and I helped out in the school holidays, and then the rule was 'the customer is always right', and leaving customers waiting unnecessarily did not happen.

In common with a lot of autistic people, I have problems understanding jokes and slang words. I remember when Rhodri was at his second residential school. I'd ring to ask how he was, and was told he was "cool" or sometimes "chilling". I wondered why they couldn't put a jumper on him. Due to the repeated use of the words, I assumed they meant something other than the obvious and looked them up on the internet for an explanation. Another confusing remark is "see you later" when you are not seeing the person later (that day) or possibly won't see them for months. A stranger I was unlikely to meet again said that to me once, and when I said "pardon" thinking I must have misheard, she repeated her remark and gave me a very peculiar look. I didn't know what to reply as I wasn't seeing her later.

People who are always say one thing, while meaning something else drives me demented! Also, people who are always 'joking'. I never know when they are joking, or being serious, and end up in total confusion. Not very long ago, someone who kept messing me about when requesting a drink, alternating between tea & coffee, came very close to having one of them poured over him! I managed to resist the temptation!

One example of a lack of understanding that I have found is that mothers of sons with Asperger's Syndrome, are often totally unable to understand my difficulties due to having the same condition. They seem unable to understand that Asperger's Syndrome is not exclusively a problem for young males. That a woman in her 50's has the same problems, seems to be totally incomprehensible to these people. Many times, such mothers have told me something along the lines of 'Pull yourself together' if I have a problem with a situation. I know that if I was to tell them to instruct their son to 'Pull himself together' when they describe some of his difficulties, then they would be extremely angry with me. So why say that to me? The people who one would think would be the most understanding, are actually the worst!

Another instance of a lack of understanding, is when people play what I call 'mind games'. To me this is a type of mental torture. I was supporting a woman in her 40's, with learning difficulties, who lived in a flat with support from agency workers. These workers complained about the woman swearing at them when she became frustrated and anxious. The agency wrote a statement for the woman to sign. The statement was along the lines of "I understand that my support worker will leave my flat for 15 minutes if I swear at them". The woman signed the statement when asked to do so. I went to visit her, after I had stopped working with her, and found the support worker sitting in his car. He said she had sworn at him, and he had left as in the agreement. She had apparently begged him not to go, but he left anyway.

Not under any such restriction myself, I went in to her to find her completely distressed, unable to understand where the support worker had gone or why she was left on her own. She had no understanding that she had 'agreed' to this action, which as far as I can see was intended as a 'punishment' for swearing. I know that I wouldn't have left her, 'punishing' an adult by adding to her anxieties and in a way that she didn't understand, was something I would not be able to do.

I can't see the problem with someone behaving as they wish in their own home. Surely that is what the rest of us do? Another woman was forced to go out for a walk to calm down, after a disagreement with a support worker who accused her of not saying "please" when asking for help in the kitchen. Does everyone always say please and thank you in their own home? I'm quite likely to say "here, hold this a minute" to Bryn, on occasions. Should I be 'punished' for this lack of courtesy? I think not.

Although physically attacking someone is naturally inadmissible, surely some normal behaviour due to being in a bad mood for any reason, is allowable. What person is happy and content all the time? We all have our bad days, when we are stressed and snap at people about us.

People should feel safe in their own homes, and should be able to live as they want to do so. That is the reason given by social services for promoting supported living.

i.e. 'People with learning difficulties can choose where to live, who to live with, and who supports them'.

This doesn't actually happen though. When Bryn left his residential college, the college and social worker wanted him to live in a supported living placement. We didn't meet the social worker until 3 months before he left college, which seemed a bit late to arrange anything.

We were told that the only other people looking for supported living, for him to share a house with, were two men in their 40's who had spent their whole lives in residential care. Bryn was 21 and lived at home, went to college and lived a very full life. Those who have spent their lives in residential care are institutionalised, would be unlikely to understand computers or want broadband internet like Bryn does. Bryn also has so much computer and TV equipment, that it generates a lot of heat. He needs two rooms (a bedroom & a living room) to himself, or a very large bedsitting room, as he has at the moment at home. This we were told was not available, he would have to watch TV in the lounge with the other residents of the house – this would definitely not suit Bryn!

I was then called to a meeting to meet the agency who would be supporting him! What about this "choose who supports you" I thought! I went along, taking my mum. The agency gave a presentation about how wonderful they thought they were. I had worked in supported living, in order to find out how it worked on the 'inside', so was able to ask some pertinent questions. I didn't pick up on the reaction of the person from the agency, but my

Mum said they had come to the meeting thinking it was a foregone conclusion, and were surprised by my grasp of the situation and that I understood what they were talking about.

Bryn, when asked where he wanted to live, said he wanted to live at home. He brought home work from college, where he had written (judging by the language this was dictated) 'I want to live in a house with other people like myself' 'I prefer to live in Bristol' etc. At the end of these pieces of work, was always the statement 'Live at (our address)'. It was easy to see that these statements were ignored by the college, as they were unadorned whereas the others had a tick by them.

Fortunately Steve had moved out of my house a few months previously, so his large bedsitting room in a ground floor extension was empty and Bryn moved in there. He and I now have a 'house share' arrangement. He lives downstairs, I live upstairs, and we share the kitchen & utility room. I do use the downstairs lounge for my craft classes, as there is no room upstairs, but only when Bryn is out. I am trying to teach him to live independently at home i.e. being able to stay by himself at times, and understanding about money, cooking simple meals etc. Then I feel, he will be able to take these skills to move into a flat on his own, to have support workers coming in and out to help him.

Often professionals have difficulty understanding the realities of having an autistic child. I remember the social worker who kept saying "I know, I know" when I tried to explain to her the inconvenience of using the toilet with Rhodri (aged 6) sitting on my lap! From conversation she turned out to be childless – little she actually knew about it!

This reminds me of a meeting I regularly attended of a network committee organised by the local council. The object of the committee was to produce a newsletter to send to all parents who had children with special needs, mostly with learning difficulties, and who lived in the council area concerned. I was the parent representative as I was the founder of a charity for children with special needs, as well as having two autistic children myself. As far as I recall, the other members included a manager of social services, a development worker for a local disability organization, a youth worker, a community nurse and someone from the council's education department. There were about 8 to 10 people in total.

I particularly remember one meeting, which sums up the attitude of professionals to those of us who have children with these difficulties. At the meeting, various members of the committee had brought articles of interest, which they thought could be included in the newsletter. One item described a government report of a change in the law relating to education, or something similar.

There was much discussion whether this item should be included. Most members of the committee were commenting that they thought it was too complicated and that "parents" wouldn't understand it or be interested in it. I was personally not interested, as I tend to follow and fight for local issues, but I knew of several of my acquaintances who did follow such national issues and would like to read about them.

Over the months, I had become very annoyed with this "Parents wouldn't be able to understand" attitude, which had been continually repeated during discussions about various subjects. When I reviewed the meetings in my head, at the end of the day, going over what was said, I decided I needed a way to point out that it wasn't the parents, but their children who had learning difficulties. I formulated a plan in my head, and waited for a suitable time to use it.

This had just occurred, so I asked the person sitting opposite me whether she had any children. I had struck unlucky, as it seemed she didn't, so I moved to the next along and asked her – she said yes. I asked another, who I seemed to remember mentioning a daughter in a previous conversation, and she said yes she had children. I said "Ah, so you are PARENTS – Do YOU understand it?" I was astounded when they said "Yes, but would parents of children with learning difficulties understand it?"

I pointed out that in the club I ran, the parents included a nursing sister, a chartered accountant, a teacher and a university lecturer, who were all a lot more qualified than me, and that if the people in the meeting could understand it, then I'm sure they could too! They said, "Surely not everyone is something like an accountant or teacher?" So, I said "No, there are some parents who have learning difficulties too, some who can't read the newsletter in the first place, and if everything is going to be at their level, then you needn't bother to produce it at all!" The article in question was published in the newsletter!

This tendency to treat parents as if they all have the difficulties of their children is something I have found time and time again, over the years. The same as, when I have told someone I have Asperger's Syndrome, they often immediately treat me as if I have a low intelligence, where actually the opposite is the case.

REACTIONS TO HEARING ABOUT MY DIAGNOSIS OF ASPERGER'S SYNDROME :

" I'm not surprised – if there is a wrong way to take something, that's the way you will take it!"

My Ex-husband

"I've known that for a long time – but I didn't like to tell you!"

My sons' Social Worker

IT WORKED FOR US!

Rhodri was incontinent until he was 7 years old. Before this he wore incontinence pads provided by the NHS. He got very hot in summer and the plastic covered 'nappies' made him get a painful rash under them.

After attending a talk by the continence nurse, I discovered that large pads were available, intended for women, that 'stuck in' to ordinary pants, and could be ordered for children of either sex. I ordered some for Rhodri and bought him some "real pants" with a TV character on, which he loved. The rash cleared as he wasn't so hot, and toilet training was easier. He wore the toddler 'pull ups' at night that have a breathable fabric rather than plastic but these were too expensive to buy for all day.

The pads needed to be changed more frequently, but we were allowed more of them, as they were less expensive, and they were easier to change than the full sized incontinence pads.

PROBLEM SOLVED !

V IS FOR VITAMINS AND DIET ETC.

It was shortly after my husband & I separated, when Bryn was 7 and Rhodri 5 years old, that talk in the autism forums on the internet was mainly about dietary interventions.

It would have been around 1998 that I heard about autistic children having improved behaviour when keeping to a gluten or casein free diet. Gluten is a substance found in wheat and casein is in milk. A GFCF (gluten free, casein free) diet was the 'in thing' to try. I had got to the stage of trying anything provided it didn't cost too much, as I was only receiving state benefits.

At that time, the University of Sunderland offered a urine test to determine whether children were likely to benefit from a GF and/or CF diet. They kindly offered to test two for the price of one for me, and after a certain difficulty (Rhodri was still wearing nappies, which made urine collection complicated) the tests showed a larger peak on the Gluten test, than the Casein test.

I tried cutting out Casein first, changing to soya milk and dairy-free cheese. These proved to taste terrible, and no discernible change was noticed in the boys' behaviour. Therefore we went back to 'normal' milk and cheese, and instead tried removing gluten from our diet. This showed a great improvement.

Bryn had for some years been suffering from a lot of bouts of diarrhoea. Mostly this would happen on a Sunday night or Monday morning. Then, due to the rule that children had to have 48 hours off school if they had diarrhoea, he was home for Monday & Tuesday. He normally didn't have another incident and I was left with a lively, perfectly healthy child to keep amused for two days! After a few occasions of this, it occurred to me that every time it was 'only him' i.e. no-one else caught this 'bug' as normally happens with stomach upsets. In the end, I decided to send him to school anyway and ignore the Monday morning diarrhoea. I would have had to lie and say he hadn't had it at home if he later had an incident in school, however this situation never occurred.

When we had gone 'gluten free', having decided that the boys were intolerant of gluten, I discovered, from his father, that Bryn had been eating three Weetabix at his house most Sundays! This confirmed the gluten intolerance as the excess wheat (Weetabix being 95% Wheat) caused his digestive system to fail and was why he got diarrhoea on Mondays!

Bryn was a lot better on a GF diet, presumably now not having stomach pains that he hadn't been able to tell me about. His digestive system recovered and several years later, when foods containing gluten were reintroduced gradually to his diet, he became able to tolerate them again. He now only avoids whole-wheat items (Weetabix, bran, wholemeal bread etc.). He eats Oatibix for breakfast, this looks like Weetabix but is made from oats which do not contain gluten.

Rhodri, however, is completely different. Gluten intolerance in his case, causes him to have episodes of extremely violent behaviour. I had always thought there was something 'odd' about the way Rhodri attacked me. One incident will always stay in my mind. I was sat in a chair in the lounge reading a book. Rhodri was sat on the floor opposite me, also looking at a book with a smile on his face, looking content. All of a sudden, completely without warning, Rhodri launched at me, growling with his eyes glazed over. He grabbed both my arms and sank his teeth into my shoulder. I had to fight him off, and try to turn him so he was facing the other way and hold his arms down by his side. He was about 5 years old. This is a sample of many hundreds of times that he has attacked me. He has been doing this since he was a baby. It was only around the time of the incident related above, that I realised when he attacked me in this sudden, extreme way (rather than the odd pinch/bite as a 'one off') his eyes went 'odd', they appeared to have a glazed over / expressionless / staring quality and I began to wonder if he was having a type of epileptic fit.

After Rhodri was eating a completely Gluten Free diet, these extreme episodes of aggression ceased. He still bit and pinched me but not to the same extent, and the 'eyes glazing over' was not happening. Unfortunately his lack of sleep, hyperactivity, need for constant care etc. meant that I continued to need regular respite care for him. I was living alone with two children who both needed 1:1 care.

Rhodri's school and respite homes were not always reliable in keeping to his diet. I remember the staff member who didn't realise that fish fingers contained gluten. She said that she didn't realise that the 'breadcrumbs' contained bread/flour and therefore gluten! When Rhodri ate foods containing gluten his behaviour became a problem.

Finally, we received funding for him to attend a residential school for children with autism. All was well for the first few months, then the GP at the school decided she would no longer prescribe gluten free food for Rhodri. The school asked me to pay, but I was not receiving any benefits for him, as he was on a residential placement paid for by the council, so Bryn & I would have to pay out of our benefits. I refused as I didn't want to use my small savings, or spend the rest of my life paying for gluten free food for Rhodri.

However, when put back onto 'normal' food, his behaviour deteriorated. He was back with his violent attacking episodes, food craving, etc. When he came home for five weeks in the summer holidays, after two half terms of 'normal' food, I decided I couldn't stand any more. I couldn't bear to watch my loving son deteriorate into a monster. So, over the school summer holidays, I 'cold-turkeyed' him from gluten. This meant suddenly removing gluten from his diet, rather than cutting down gradually, which causes less of a problem. This is the same as when drug addicts stop taking drugs, in fact gluten is a drug to people like Rhodri.

It was during this period that I suffered so many bruises from bites and pinches on my arms, that it was impossible to see skin colour, only various shades of purple, green and yellow as I had bruises on top of bruises. I couldn't even go to the doctors to get my injuries documented as various people suggested. Other patients in the waiting room would have been at risk, as I would have had to take Rhodri with me. Rhodri was excluded from one of his respite homes because of his extremely violent behaviour, but within 3 weeks, the gluten was out of his system and he was greatly improved, stopped food craving and attacked me less often.

Towards the end of the holidays, with the help of my Mum, who had Bryn to stay while Rhodri was home from school, I baked vast quantities of gluten free bread, biscuits and cake. These I froze and took them back to school with Rhodri. I told them that I couldn't stand what they had done to my son, that he was back on a gluten free diet and that I would pay! I would go short of food myself rather than have Rhodri suffer from his gluten intolerance. I had taken enough food for a couple of weeks to allow them time to purchase the right foods. <u>I was never asked for money!</u> Presumably, the difference in the child I returned to them, rather than the child they sent home, meant that they realised Rhodri's need for gluten free food. The deterioration of his behaviour when they introduced gluten was slower to show a difference, but the great improvement in his behaviour when I returned him to school, made the GP change her mind and prescribe gluten free food again.

Other than gluten, the foods to which Rhodri is intolerant have changed over the years. He was only 3 years old when I realised that oranges and chocolate 'set him off' i.e. he became unmanageable and attacked me. Later, it was apples and salted crisps. At this point, Walkers started making 'salt & shake crisps', which was great as Rhodri could have crisps without the salt. Unfortunately, I found a carer teaching him how to open the salt packet! However, his intolerances changed later and he can now eat crisps, apples and oranges, but he still has to avoid milk & plain chocolate, lemons and vinegar. He has always been able to eat white chocolate without problems. He is also intolerant to artificial colours, flavours and preservatives, so even the ingredients on gluten free food has to be checked to see if it contains anything artificial.

My sons are now both taking Omega-3 fish oils and zinc citrate. The zinc was suggested by a homeopathic therapist as being good for 'the teenage years'. I'm more aware of how they help Bryn, as Rhodri is in 24 hour, 52 week care. Bryn is calmer when he is taking his supplements and the zinc seems to improve his sociability. It is noticeable when we run out, as he is less 'eager to please' on these occasions. Then when the new order comes, he improves again. He also takes Kalms each morning, which seems to take the 'edge' off his anxiety issues.

W is for Worrying

Most autistic people are good at worrying!

What time is right? How do I do that? Who do I speak to? What time to ring someone? Worry, Worry, Worry

I have always said that if 'worrying' was an Olympic sport – I would get a gold medal!

When I have been employed and had done something wrong, I was always worried that I would get sacked. It isn't easy to explain, it's not a general "I'm worried" worry. It's an all encompassing worry – the same worry going round and round, over and over in my head. I remember several times when I had done something wrong at work and became so scared of someone finding out, that I was terrified to go to work the next morning. I was persuaded to go by my husband, and when I got there the manager said "That's ok, easily sorted" or something like that. This, or something like it, has happened many times. I'm always surprised that errors can be taken so lightly.

I find it's difficult to know whether or not I am 'overstaying my welcome' when visiting a new friend, or even an old one for that matter – on the occasions I actually have one. Does an invitation for a cup of tea mean the time it takes to drink one (about 10 – 15 mins)? I try to keep to one hour, which I thought would be a good period – some people say "pop round for an hour". The trouble with that is I tend to keep looking at my watch to make sure I don't stay too long, and I get funny looks and people say "Do you have to be somewhere?" Of course, it's easier if there is a clock in the room! My usual learning routine, of trying to imagine myself in the other person's place doesn't work for this, as the only people who come to my home are people who are paid to do so (e.g. social workers, support workers) or those who come to a craft club I run, which has set times. It's easier to stay home alone really!

A while ago I supported a gentleman with learning difficulties, who would beat me to the Gold medal at the 'worrying' Olympics. I tried to remember my worst times of worrying, to work out how I stopped, in order to help him to do the same. The main thing for me was to go out and find people to talk to, even if only shop assistants at the till. This gives my brain a break in its circle of confusion.

I have found learning Reiki beneficial. Doing a Reiki energy meditation is very calming, and gives me something else to think about. The routine of meditating every day before bedtime is helpful and calms my mind for sleep.

X IS FOR XMAS

Christmas is a very confusing time for autistic children especially. Everything seems to be changes. The house looks different with Christmas Decorations, especially if parents take the opportunity to put them up when their children are out or in bed! I remember when Rhodri was moving from his residential school to his care home. The manager remarked that his trial visits had better not be during the two weeks over Christmas, or he may think that the paper chains were permanent fixtures at the home.

Many years, for my children and me, Christmas was not really different to any other day. Well, we went to my parents for lunch every Sunday, so it was like a Sunday mostly on a different day. Until Rhodri moved to 52 week care, aged about 12, Christmas Day involved walking the streets for an hour two or three times a day, just like any other day. He didn't understand why the shops were shut, and there was nowhere to go, except to walk. When he started at the residential 52-week school, he only came home on Sundays, and I didn't confuse him by taking him home for lunch on Christmas Day, if it didn't fall on the right day of the week.

As younger children, neither Bryn nor Rhodri liked opening parcels. They didn't seem to understand that there was something nice inside. They were not interested in a cube shape object decorated with Christmas Trees etc. I had to open all their presents, and even when showed what was inside they often gave it back to me because it was new and not familiar. I just took to leaving the items round the house, as soon they would be familiar looking and would be played with by one or other of the boys. It is very difficult buying presents, when their interests were so far behind their chronological years. I remember when Bryn asked for Harry Potter Pyjamas, he was about 16 years old and they only went up to age 12! I bought a t-shirt with Harry Potter, cut out the motif, and sewed it onto a pair of pyjamas his size.

Bryn always screamed at the suggestion to hang up a stocking, place one on his bed, or even to leave it outside the door. I left a filled one, but he wouldn't open it. I always loved having a stocking from Father Christmas when I was a child, and was upset that neither of my sons were interested in stockings when they were small. I hated listening to mothers discussing how their children love their presents and about seeing them open them, as I felt I missed out on this.

Bryn suddenly became interested in Father Christmas at the age of 12 years. That year we went round to visit all the Santa's we could find, as I felt I was making up for missing out on this magical time for so long. It looked a bit odd, as he was twice as tall as all the other children in the queue, but he didn't seem to mind, and I was past caring.

From that year, Bryn's understanding of Father Christmas bringing presents grew. He gradually learnt to ask for the gifts he wanted. Now, aged 23, he writes his wish list for

Father Christmas. I've just been given one, and it is the middle of July. He knows that he has to wait until 25th December for the gifts to come.

Over the years they have also learnt to unwrap presents. When they were small, I used to give them their gifts unwrapped, or just in a carrier bag, as I had to unwrap the ones from other people. Now they seem to enjoy tearing off the wrapping paper like anyone else.

My own problem with Christmas is that I'm happy and looking forward to it during the autumn months. I make lots of gifts to sell on my craft stalls from September to early December. But a couple of weeks before the big day, I get anxious and dread the day arriving. I wish that I could just go away somewhere on my own, and not have Christmas. I'm the same with going away on holiday, I look forward to it, tell everyone I'm going away, then a few days before I don't want to go. If it was left to me, we wouldn't go, but Bryn isn't like me – he is awake early eager for the activity, so whether it's Christmas Day or our holiday, I just have to make the best of things. I think trying to please Brynmor, and my Mum & Dad all together adds to the stress.

I was always ill at Christmas as a child. Normally getting a stomach upset a day or two before. I remember never being able to eat much Christmas Dinner because I was suffering from diarrhoea, and my Mum usually accused me of doing this every year on purpose!

"SILVER LININGS"

The proverb says "Every Cloud has a Silver Lining".

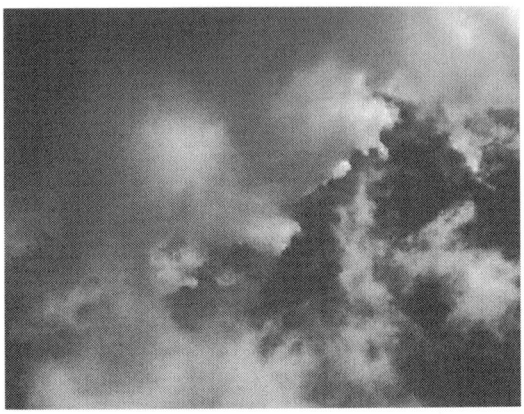

Although it can be difficult, I try to find the 'Silver Linings' to having two autistic children when I can, for example:

You don't have to struggle through rain, wind or snow to take them to school. Just walk to the garden gate (sometimes in dressing gown & slippers) and put them in a taxi or minibus!
(school transport provided by the council)

You will never lose your bunch of keys
(A RADAR key is about 4 inches long!)

You don't have the embarrassment of your children making comments such as "Mummy, why is that lady so fat?" (assuming they are non-verbal, like mine)

Y IS FOR YOU

This chapter consists of two true stories I wrote.

"YOU WILL HAVE A GREAT TIME, IT'S WONDERFUL, SO RELAXING"

My sons' social worker had been trying to persuade me, as a carer, to go to a local relaxation day provided by a charity. I had been refusing to go, as I had no-one to go with me. Finally, in order to stop her repeated requests, I booked a place for this day which, I was told, was wonderful with a lovely lunch, and all for free!

So I went to the large house, run by the charity. I arrived first, as usual, and was followed soon after by other carers – two groups of two friends and one group of three. One of the groups of two obviously knew me from somewhere – they were 'ringing a bell' in my head, but I couldn't remember who they were, and where I knew them from. They were obviously hostile towards me, staring, pointing & giggling, more like they were in junior school, and didn't speak to me, so I decided to ignore their behaviour and hopefully not show them I had noticed.

So, there I was as usual – on my own, when everyone else had a friend to talk to. The facilitator explained the layout of the rooms. She then disappeared, just as I was thinking perhaps she would talk to me. I went into the 'art room', where art materials were left around to use. I was made to feel very unwelcome by the 'group of 3' who acted like they had booked the room, and had moved most of the materials to their table. – I went out.

The other room had a drama/dance type activity, not really something in my line. I tried to join in with this, but the giggling duo were in there, so I wandered outside. Here I did find someone to talk to for a few minutes, discussing the roses with the gardener, but he had work to do.

I thought I might as well stay for this "lovely lunch" I had heard about. So I sat in the garden bored, with nothing to do, on my own for about an hour. The lunch turned out to be pasta or curry, both of which I dislike. After a slice of bread and butter, I went home in tears.

I didn't see what was so lovely about being excluded for being on my own, and this was the very reason I had not wanted to go. It only accentuates the fact I have no friends. I try to choose the carer's activities I attend, with care, as this situation (although normally without the giggling) otherwise continually repeats itself. The social worker said she couldn't understand it, when she asked me how I got on, she had had a wonderful time when she went. Fortunately, each carer could only attend this 'relaxation day' once, so I wasn't made to go again.

" YOU WEREN'T IN ! "

Remarked in an accusing tone by the delivery person from the local pharmacist, attached to the doctor's surgery. It is a remark that I have heard many times, after my friend, Steve, who lived in my house for a while, became paraplegic and a permanent wheelchair user.

The rest of the world, seemed to think that this meant he, and I, were confined to the house for the rest of our days, except when visiting the doctor or hospital. Why should he, as a disabled person want to go out? they seemed to be saying.

The district nurse had called the day previously, and decided without telling us to order something from the pharmacist for Steve, and told them to deliver it. We were out when it arrived, not having any idea it was coming, and in any case, having previously arranged with the surgery that we would collect any prescriptions. I didn't want to stay in all day, every day, just to answer the door. Things had previously got to a head, when the delivery person – finding us out one day when we weren't expecting him – had tipped all the tablets into the paper bag, and put them through the letterbox as the bottle wouldn't fit! On the occasion at the top of the page, he had had to come back as the item wouldn't fit through the letterbox at all.

I had already had to 'train' the district nurse to phone to say when she would be arriving to change Steve's catheter. We were told the day, but no idea of time, and I refused to stay in the house all day, and Steve having to stay waiting in bed, if she wasn't actually coming until the afternoon. We were told that no-one else minded. Presumably people who worked didn't mind having to take a day off every six weeks or so, for this necessary procedure. After a couple of times when I was out, they phoned in the morning to tell me where we were on the list, to give an indication of when they would be coming. I don't know if other people now receive this information, or if they are still kept in bed all day.

The same assumption was normal when my children were small. Why should someone want to go out with two autistic children?? Apparently I should confine myself to the house. When Rhodri was diagnosed autistic, so we knew that both my sons had the disability, someone told me "You won't be able to go out at all now"! I took no notice. Actually, staying in was hell – we only had a small house and garden, no room to run round to get exercise. We were mostly out, walking, bus rides, train rides, car rides. Going shopping, to parks, to playgrounds, to the seaside… I wasn't going to let my children's autism stop them from having a 'normal' childhood, being able to go out on trips.

Z IS FOR ZZZZ (SLEEPING)

I can't remember having a particular problem sleeping when I was young. I used to lie in bed and go into one of my imaginary worlds, which I wrote about earlier in the book. My sleeping problems started when I had my children.

Bryn slept the most of first 24 hours of his life, midwives kept coming to give him a heel-prick test and went away as he was asleep! However, he seemed to think that was enough sleep for a life-time, as he went on to sleep hardly at all. I remember midwives etc saying "he must sleep more than you say" (about 8 hours a day), they treated me as if I was stupid, so I made a chart and shaded all the time he was asleep (about 8 hours in 24) and it was in about 2 hour slots!

When Rhodri came along, I learnt what other mums had meant when they said they put their babies down to sleep, if I ever put Bryn down he would scream! I tried the leaving him to scream method, but after an hour I couldn't take any more of it. He used to lie in my bed with me – my husband worked nights, so there was plenty of room and he didn't need to be where I might roll on him. When Rhodri was due, I had to get him to sleep in his own bed.

First I put him in his bed and laid down with him until he went to sleep, then I put a pillow by the side of him (the other side was by the wall) and pillows on the floor in case he fell out. This was fine for a while, until he decided for some reason that he didn't want to sleep in his bed. He slept on the floor, just behind the closed door, so I couldn't open it without banging his head! After a couple of nights, I realised I had to stop him doing this and to sleep in his bed. I noticed he had dragged a blanket down to lie on, so I put the blanket slightly away from the door with a pillow and put him to sleep there. After a couple of nights like that, I moved the blanket slightly nearer the bed, and so on until it was just beside the bed. Then I put the mattress on the floor beside the bed, where the blanket had been the night before. A few days later, I put the mattress back on the bed base and he was sleeping in his bed again!

Rhodri, however, was different again. He was always coming into my bed, usually because he had wet his! I was tired all the time, as Bryn was awake until 1am and Rhodri usually woke at 4 or 5am, although he has been known to be awake for nearly 36 hours without a sleep. Many nights I had to take Rhodri for a walk up and down outside the house in the early hours of the morning, as he wasn't tired to sleep, and kept running round the house. The fresh air often helped him feel sleepy again, and he would go back to sleep. I couldn't drop off then, as I had been having cups of tea to keep me awake for hours. I found out about Melatonin on the internet and ordered it from the USA – this helped Rhodri go to sleep, but not necessarily stay asleep. He was later prescribed this and other sedatives, by his psychiatrist, which we alternated as he seemed to become immune to them after a while.

Rhodri needed lots of exercise to get him tired, and still does for that matter. When my sons were young, I always had tea ready when they got home from school, as I couldn't cook with them there. I was a lone parent by this time. Then we went out for a walk, for at least an hour. If it poured with rain, we went to a supermarket instead, or the Mall (an undercover shopping centre) where they enjoyed walking up and down in the dry. In the school holidays, we had two or three long walks of about an hour every day, to get Rhodri tired. I would sometimes walk to my Mum's, leave Bryn there (who didn't like all the walking) and walk Rhodri the long way round to go home. My Dad would bring Bryn back in the car later.

In those days I didn't live – I existed! I was permanently tired. The years are a bit of a blur now, all my time was spent trying to keep my children occupied and safe, and fighting for a residential placement for Rhodri.

Rhodri moved to a 38 week residential school when he was 7 years old, and to a 52 week placement four years later.

Strangely, Bryn sleeps more now that he is an adult. He normally goes to bed about 10 - 11pm, depending what time he has to get up in the morning. He gets up at 7am on the days he goes to Work Training, and 8am on other days. He is busy most days, and as his work training is at a farm, he gets a lot of fresh air and exercise.

USEFUL WEBSITES
(Including the ones mentioned in this book)

National Autistic Society   www.autism.org.uk

Crelling Safety Harnesses   www.crelling.com

Safe Shield Ltd   www.safeshield-ltd.co.uk

RADAR   www.radar.org.uk

My Craft site: www.lynnescrafts.blogspot.co.uk

My Reiki site: www.spiritcraftreiki.blogspot.co.uk

This book's website: ww.AtoZaspergers.blogspot.co.uk
(Including autism badges, hats, etc)

While at Oakwood Court College, Bryn was filmed using computer avatars as an aid to communication. The project, undertaken by K.C. Kelly-Marwick, and consisting of several videos of Bryn using an avatar with a webcam, can be seen at the following website:

http://archive.excellencegateway.org.uk/page.aspx?o=265496

It is hoped that research will continue in order to improve communication for autistic people by the use of computers.

THE END AND THE FUTURE

I started this book, as I mentioned before, after listening to a talk about teaching social skills to autistic children with challenging behaviour. It has taken about 8 years to write, as I did a few chapters, put it away, then a year or so later, got it out again, etc. This time I got it out, I was surprised by how much I had changed in my conversational abilities etc. I had to go through and put a lot of statements in the past tense, as I no longer have so many problems with social matters.

I hope to continue to spread the message that having Autism isn't the end of world, that autistic people have a lot to offer, and have a right to be accepted as themselves.

I am now self-employed, and also care for Bryn, who lives in a bedsitting room in an extension of our family home. I find self-employment doesn't have the same anxieties that having an employer does. I make and sell novelty gifts from September to Christmas, run a craft group for carers, teach craft parties and give talks and demonstrations to groups such as the Women's Institute.

I am also starting to teach Reiki healing and provide treatments as I am qualified as a Reiki Master Teacher. I would particularly like to teach people with Asperger's Syndrome, or other disabled people, and their carers, as Reiki is a wonderful way to relax and feel calm.

Printed in Great Britain
by Amazon.co.uk, Ltd.,
Marston Gate.